PHARMACEUTICAL TECHNOLOGY
Drug Stability

ELLIS HORWOOD BOOKS IN BIOLOGICAL SCIENCES
General Editor: Dr. Alan Wiseman, Department of Biochemistry, University of Surrey, Guildford

SERIES IN PHARMACEUTICAL TECHNOLOGY
Editor: Professor M. H. RUBINSTEIN, School of Health Sciences, Liverpool Polytechnic

MICROBIAL QUALITY ASSURANCE IN PHARMACEUTICALS, COSMETICS AND TOILETRIES
Edited by S. Bloomfield *et al.*

DRUG MONITORING*
Edited by S. H. Curry

PHARMACEUTICAL THERMAL ANALYSIS*
J. L. Ford and P. Timmins

TABLET MACHINE INSTRUMENTATION IN PHARMACEUTICS
P. Ridgway Watt

PHARMACEUTICAL CHEMISTRY, Volume 1 Drug Synthesis
Professor Dr. H. J. Roth *et al.*

PHARMACEUTICAL CHEMISTRY, Volume 2 Drug Analysis*
Professor Dr. H. J. Roth *et al.*

PHARMACEUTICAL TECHNOLOGY: Controlled Drug Release, Volume 1
Edited by M. H. Rubinstein

PHARMACEUTICAL TECHNOLOGY: Controlled Drug Release, Volume 2*
Edited by M. H. Rubinstein

PHARMACEUTICAL TECHNOLOGY: Tableting Technology, Volume 1
Edited by M. H. Rubinstein

PHARMACEUTICAL TECHNOLOGY: Tableting Technology, Volume 2*
Edited by M. H. Rubinstein

PHARMACEUTICAL TECHNOLOGY: Drug Stability*
Edited by M. H. Rubinstein

PHARMACEUTICAL TECHNOLOGY: Drug Targeting*
Edited by M. H. Rubinstein

UNDERSTANDING BACTERIAL RESISTANCE
D. A. Russell and I. Chopra

RADIOPHARMACEUTICALS IN MEDICINE
A. Theobald

PHARMACEUTICAL PREFORMULATION:
The Physicochemical Properties of Drug Substances
J. I. Wells

* In preparation

PHARMACEUTICAL
TECHNOLOGY
Drug Stability

Editor:

M. H. RUBINSTEIN, B.Pharm., Ph.D., M.R.Pharm.S., M.I.Chem.E., C.Eng.
Professor of Pharmaceutical Technology
School of Health Sciences, Liverpool Polytechnic

ELLIS HORWOOD LIMITED
Publishers · Chichester

Halsted Press: a division of
JOHN WILEY & SONS
New York · Chichester · Brisbane · Toronto

First published in 1989 by
ELLIS HORWOOD LIMITED
Market Cross House, Cooper Street,
Chichester, West Sussex, PO19 1EB, England
The publisher's colophon is reproduced from James Gillison's drawing of the ancient Market Cross, Chichester.

Distributors:

Australia and New Zealand:
JACARANDA WILEY LIMITED
GPO Box 859, Brisbane, Queensland 4001, Australia
Canada:
JOHN WILEY & SONS CANADA LIMITED
22 Worcester Road, Rexdale, Ontario, Canada
Europe and Africa:
JOHN WILEY & SONS LIMITED
Baffins Lane, Chichester, West Sussex, England
North and South America and the rest of the world:
Halsted Press: a division of
JOHN WILEY & SONS
605 Third Avenue, New York, NY 10158, USA
South-East Asia
JOHN WILEY & SONS (SEA) PTE LIMITED
37 Jalan Pemimpin # 05–04
Block B, Union Industrial Building, Singapore 2057
Indian Subcontinent
WILEY EASTERN LIMITED
4835/24 Ansari Road
Daryaganj, New Delhi 110002, India

© 1989 M. H. Rubinstein/Ellis Horwood Limited

British Library Cataloguing in Publication Data
Pharmaceutical technology.
1. Drugs. Stability. For pharmaceutics
I. Rubinstein, M. H. (Michael Henry), *1944–*
615′.19

Library of Congress CIP data available

ISBN 0–7458–0344–X (Ellis Horwood Limited)
ISBN 0–470–21411–2 (Halsted Press)

Typeset in Times by Ellis Horwood Limited
Printed in Great Britain by Hartnolls, Bodmin

Table of contents

Preface

Pharmaceutical technology is the science of producing acceptable dosage forms which once administered, release the drug substance into the body at a predetermined time and rate. However, the dosage forms should also be stable and continue to release the drug at the same time and rate even after prolonged ageing. No measurable chemical or physical degradation must occur. The problems of producing dosage forms that are stable and remain so under differing climatic conditions is a science in itself and this third volume from a 'series within a series' is designed to reflect new advances and techniques for enhancing drug stability from formulated pharmaceuticals. It represents a range of highly topical areas from authors of international repute.

Cyclodextrins have been used for many years to form inclusion compounds with a variety of drug molecules. The first chapter presents a comprehensive review of the current areas that cyclodextrins have in modern pharmaceutical formulation. They can enhance the thermal and oxidative stability of drug molecules and in some instances hydrolysis can be reduced. Inclusion compounds may also improve drug dissolution rate and increase drug absorption through biological membranes. So cyclodextrins are exciting and important compounds which will obviously play a very important role in pharmaceutical formulation in the 1990s.

Liposomes have attracted a lot of interest in recent years as unique drug carrier systems. In the second chapter liposomes have been used to stabilize local anaesthetics and the degradation kinetics evaluated, whilst in Chapter 3 the processing factors influencing the stability of freeze-dried sodium ethacrynate have been investigated. Later chapters look at the use of colloidal and porous silica as carriers and stabilizing systems in solid, semi-solid and liquid dosage forms. New analytical techniques have not been ignored and in Chapter 9 the advantage in terms of selectivity, time saving and economy of using short and ultra-short HPLC columns for drug analysis in dissolution testing, is presented. Finally in Chapter 12 a control system is described for monitoring changes in particle growth by crystallization in pharmaceutical suspensions.

As with the predecessor volumes (*Tableting Technology*, Volume 1, and *Controlled drug release*, Volume 1, published by Ellis Horwood Ltd in 1987), the book is based on contributions made to the prestigious series of annual conferences held to review progress in pharmaceutical technology on a worldwide basis. This volume includes all the latest developments, incorporating international discussion from Harrogate (1986), Canterbury (1987) and London (1988).

August 1988

Michael H. Rubinstein

1

Cyclodextrins, their value in pharmaceutical technology

D. Duchêne, C. Vaution and F. Glomot
Laboratoire de Pharmacie Galénique et Biopharmacie, Faculté de
Pharmacie de Paris-Sud, Rue Jean Baptiste Clément, 92290 Chatenay
Malabry, France

SUMMARY

Cyclodextrins are cyclic oligosaccharides consisting of a variable number of
glucose units (usually 6 to 8). The ring formed by cyclodextrins is externally
very hydrophilic and relatively apolar internally. In liquid or solid medium,
these molecules are capable of forming inclusion compounds with many
other molecules. The inclusion compounds thus formed display interesting
properties and may increase the stability of the guest molecules. Greater
stability may be shown towards heat, resulting in lower volatility or higher
thermal resistance. In addition, greater stability towards oxidation may
result. It may also be important for products in solution, since in certain
cases, hydrolysis is inhibited to varying degrees.

For relatively insoluble active ingredients, inclusion may improve the
solubility or drug dissolution rate. Depending on the stability constant of the
inclusion compound formed, a better passage of the active ingredient
through membranes may be observed. *In vivo*, this may be reflected by an
increase in bioavailability, with a simultaneous increase in therapeutic
effectiveness.

INTRODUCTION

Cyclodextrins have been known for nearly a century and have been isolated
by Villiers [1] in 1981 from the degradation products of starch. The
description of their preparation, isolation and main characteristics was made
by Schardinger in the years 1903 to 1911 [2–4].

Cyclodextrins and inclusion compounds

Cyclodextrins are cyclic oligosaccharides produced by the enzymatic degradation of starch. The enzyme, cyclodextrin glycosyl transferase, is produced by different bacilli, especially *Bacillus macerans*. Depending on the reaction conditions, cyclodextrins contain six, seven or eight glucose units, connected by α-(1,4) bonds, known as α-, β- and γ-cyclodextrins. The particular form of the molecule requires a special arrangement of the different functional groups. Generally the interior of the cyclodextrin cavity is apolar in relation to water, and the exterior is hydrophilic.

Table 1 — Properties of the main cyclodextrins

Cyclodextrin	No. of glucoses	Molecular weight	Solubility in water (g/100 cm^3)	Cavity dimensions (Å)		
				Depth	i.d.	o.d.
α-cyclohexaamylose	6	972	14.50	7.9–8.0	4.7–5.2	14.6±0.4
β-cyclohexaamylose	7	1135	1.85	7.9–8.0	6.0–6.4	15.4±0.4
γ-cyclohexaamylose	8	1297	23.20	7.9–8.0	7.5–8.3	17.5±0.4

Some of the properties of cyclodextrins are given in Table 1. Cyclodextrins are water-soluble; β-cyclodextrin being the least soluble. Solubility increases sharply with temperature, allowing easy recrystallization on cooling.

One of the most interesting properties of cyclodextrins is their ability to form inclusion compounds with a wide variety of molecules, which apparently only have to satisfy a single condition: namely to be adaptable entirely, or at least partially, to the cavity of the cyclodextrins [5]. Inclusion compounds are usually prepared in a liquid medium.

In the case of water-soluble materials, a drug is added to an aqueous solution of cyclodextrin, usually in stoichiometric quantities. The mixture is heated with agitation for several hours, or even several days. The inclusion formed precipitates spontaneously or by cooling. The water solubility of the drug can very often be increased by incorporating a suitable additive [6,7]. The mixture can also be freeze-dried or spray-dried [6,8–10]. The final product in this case is amorphous.

If the substance to be included is insoluble in water, it is dissolved in an organic solvent and added, with agitation, to a hot aqueous solution of cyclodextrin. Crystallization takes place within hours or days.

In some cases, the formation of the complex in the solid phase is thermodynamically spontaneous, although its stability is greater in aqueous solution than in the solid phase [11]. Inclusion is normally achieved by microgrinding [11,12].

The inclusion of a drug molecule in a cyclodextrin molecule consititutes a true molecular micro-encapsulation that is likely to alter the physicochemical and even the biological properties of the drug molecule considerably. This has encouraged research into application in the area of formulation. In Japan, these investigations culminated in the marketing of a prostaglandin E_2/β-cyclodextrin complex, Prostarmon, marketed by Ono [13].

At the pharmacological technological level, the applications of inclusions are essentially in the improvement of molecule stability [14] and, above all, the improvement of their solubility and bioavailability [15].

Improved stability
The improvement of stability may have three essential objectives: heat stability, oxidation resistance and hydrolysis resistance (or stability in aqueous solution).

Heat stability
Substances included in cyclodextrins to improve their stability may be liquid or solid.

Reduction of volatility
The reduction of volatility can be demonstrated by a rise in the boiling point or evaporation conditions of the liquids, or of sublimation for solids. Szejtli [16–20] prepared inclusion compounds with many volatile substances, including spices, plant flavours and essences, camphor, menthol and thymol. The inclusion compounds obtained facilitated the handling of the products, particularly as they transform a liquid into solid. The volatility of the substances produced is sharply reduced, and this has been closely investigated with anethole [16].

The value of these inclusions is to permit improvements in the quality of the pharmaceutical dosage forms in which they are incorporated, especially suppositories [18,19] and inhalations [17,20]. In suppositories, their melting point and hardness are often lowered by adding volatile substances, and the incorporation of these substances as inclusions often overcomes these drawbacks [19]. In the case of inhalations containing high proportions of volatile essences, the preparation is liquid, difficult to handle, and is sometimes volatilized too rapidly if mixed with boiling water. By solidifying the product, inclusion facilitates handling and slows down its vaporization while at this same time prolonging its effect [20].

The reduction of volatility can be examined by differential thermal analysis or by thermogravimetry. These techniques were used by Uekama for inclusions of clofibrate in β-cyclodextrin [21], cinnamic acid in β-cyclodextrin [22], and benzaldehyde in α-, β- and γ-cyclodextrins [23]. Nakai *et al.* [24] used thermogravimetry to analyse inclusions of parahydroxybenzoic acid in α- and β-cyclodextrins. The sublimation of parahydroxybenzoic acid at 180°C and 210°C is considerably reduced, particularly with α-cyclodextrin, and this is probably due to a closer adjustment of the molecule in the α-cyclodextrin cavity than in that of β-cyclodextrin.

An interesting stabilization effect achieved by inclusion in β-cyclodextrin, is that of the 5-mononitrate of isosorbid [25]. This is a volatile substance, and, during the storage of tablets, needles are formed at the surface, especially at certain temperatures and humidities. An inclusion eliminates this process and also reduces the degradation of the product with time.

Higher heat resistance

In the same way that inclusion raises the boiling point and evaporation and sublimation temperatures, it can also raise the melting point. This has been observed for metronidazole included in β-cyclodextrin [26] and for prostaglandin F_{2_a} [27]. Another demonstration of higher heat resistance is the elevation of the decomposition temperature. Szejtli investigated a series of aromatic oils [16]. In the case of essence of marjoram, for example, the volatile compounds are liberated and can be identified by thin film chromatography above 100°C in the case of the pure product, or in the form of a physical mixture with β-cyclodextrin, with their decomposition occurring at 240°C. If inclusion is carried out, the volatile substances only appear above 160°C, and decomposition only takes place above 300°C.

Oxidation resistance

Oxygen

The protective action of complex formation with cyclodextrins can be investigated by placing the products to be tested in a Warburg apparatus, under oxygen, at 37°C. The absorption of oxygen is measured at regular time intervals.

Using this method, Szejtli [28,29] showed an improvement in the stability of vitamin D_3, when it is complexed with β-cyclodextrin. From these results, it would appear that pure vitamin D_3 can fix 140 µl/mg of oxygen, and that the physical mixture is worse than this. However, the inclusion complex fixed only 11.2% of this amount over the same experimental time period (500 h).

Szejtli [16] used the same method to study the oxidation resistance of vegetable essences complexed with β-cyclodextrin.

Oxidation accelerators

Heat, light and metal salts (copper sulphate) all increase the degradation of vitamin D_3 by oxidation. This can be inhibited, and considerably reduced, by inclusion of the vitamin in β-cyclodextrin [28,29]. The product so treated can be presented in tablet form, having better stability against heat than tablets of the pure vitamin [28,29]. The complex vitamin D_3/β-cyclodextrin preserves 94% of its therapeutic activity, even after being stored for seven days at 60°C [30]. Similarly, the inclusion of vitamin A in α-cyclodextrin increases its stability against heat [31]. The sensitivity to light of clofibrate [21] and guaiazulene [32] is reduced by inclusion in β- and γ-cylodextrins.

Resistance to hydrolysis and to degradation in solution

The foregoing results tend to imply that the inclusion of a drug molecule in cyclodextrin generally imparts good stability to the molecule. In actual fact, this is not always the case, especially for stability in aqueous medium. Many molecules have been investigated, and the results vary considerably depending on the drug molecule, the type of cyclodextrin employed, and the pH of the medium. A number of results are reviewed below, to show this diversity.

The stability of vitamin K_3 inclusions in solution, investigated by Szejtli [33] is poor irrespective of the pH, and β-cyclodextrin actually accelerates decomposition. Møllgaard Andersen and Bundgaard showed that the degradation of hydrocortisone in β-cyclodextrin is accelerated in alkaline medium, whereas it is virtually unchanged in a neutral or acidic media [34]. This can be explained by the degradation mode of hydrocortisone, which is different in alkaline and acid media. These authors [35] further investigated the stability of betamethasone 17-valerate in aqueous alkaline solution, in which this drug undergoes a rearrangement into the less active 21-valerate. While α-cyclodextrin has no effect on this rearrangement, β-cyclodextrin was found to accelerate it, and γ-cyclodextrin slowed it down substantially. These results are explained by the differences of conformation of the inclusion compounds (1/1) formed. With nitrazepam, Møllgaard Andersen and Bundgaard [36] also showed that the presence of β-cyclodextrin has no effect on hydrolysis in 0.1 M hydrochloric acid medium. This could have been due to the ionization of the nitrazepam at this pH, since the ionized products do not easily form inclusions with cyclodextrins.

Various investigations have been conducted with aspirin. Nakai and Terada [12,37], examining its stability in the solid state, associated with α-, β- and γ-cyclodextrins, in the form of inclusions, physical mixtures, or ground mixtures, showed that, if the acetoxyl groups are free, the molecule is relatively stable, and if they are connected by hydrogen bonds to the hydroxyl groups of the cyclodextrins, the aspirin molecule becomes unstable.

Nakai [23] investigated the hydrolysis of aspirin at pH 1.0 in the presence of α-, β- and γ-cyclodextrins. The degradation constant does not vary in the presence of α-cyclodextrin, but is reduced with β- and γ-cyclodextrins; the effect of β-cyclodextrin being more pronounced. This is owing to the impossibility of including aspirin in α-cyclodextrin, of its good inclusion in β-cyclodextrin, and its excessively loose inclusion in γ-cyclodextrin, leaving a void into which a proton or molecule of water can penetrate.

The results of work on indomethacin are contradictory. Szejtli [38], reported that inclusion in β-cyclodextrin does not protect indomethacin from degradation at pH 8.0. However in a patent, the Sumimoto Chemical company reports a stabilizing effect of the inclusion [39], and Hamada [40] confirmed this result, suggesting also that the addition of α-cyclodextrin has no effect.

For barbiturates, Nagai [41] reported that the degradation of hexobarbital in alkaline solution at pH 12 is increased by β-cyclodextrin and slightly decreased by α- and γ-cyclodextrins. Min [42] and Kyoko [43] reported an improvement in the stability of aqueous solutions of phenobarbital and various barbiturates by the addition of β-cyclodextrin. Fujioka [44] investigated the degradation of bencyclane in acidic medium and showed that its inclusion caused a reduction in degradation, dependent on the cyclodextrin used; the rising rank order being α, γ and β.

Proscillaridin is unstable in gastric medium. Uekama [45] showed that inclusions in α-, β- and γ-cyclodextrins reduce the instability at pH 1.46 at 37°C. However, this result is only really significant with β- and γ-cyclodextrins, since the α cavity is too small and cannot protect the proscillaridin.

According to Møllgaard Andersen and Bundgaard [26], the hydrolysis of metronidazole benzoate is reduced by inclusion in β-cyclodextrin, and the inclusion also appears to slow down the growth of crystals in suspension.

Many patents, particularly Japanese, report the inclusion of prostaglandins in α- and β-cyclodextrins, as well as their methylated derivatives [46–52]. Although their interpretation is often difficult, an improvement in stability generally appears to be the case in aqueous solutions, as well as in the storage of freeze-dried products. Uekama [53] showed that the inclusion of prostaglandin E_1 in γ-cyclodextrin increased its heat stability and slowed down its conversion to prostaglandin A_1.

Many other substances have also been investigated, including ampicillin and methicillin, whose hydrolysis rates were significantly decreased by inclusion in β-cyclodextrin [54]. Similarly, the presence of β-cyclodextrin slows down the degradation of cinnarizine in acidic solution [55].

Improved dissolution and bioavailability
In vitro *investigations, higher water solubility*
Demonstration of the effect of cyclodextrins
Hamada *et al.* [40] studied the influence of α- and β-cyclodextrins on the solubility of a series of non-steroidal anti-inflammatory substances, by comparing it with that of glucose. For these products, glucose appears to have no effect, α-cyclodextrin is either ineffective or only slightly effective, and β-cyclodextrin causes an increase in solubility. These results are explained by the formation of inclusion compounds, in accordance with the size of the drug molecules in comparison with the dimensions of the cyclodextrin cavity.

It is unnecessary for the inclusion to be preformed for higher solubility to occur. This was shown by Corrigan and Stanley, working on phenobarbitone [56], and on benzothiazide derivatives [57]. In both cases, simple physical mixtures of the active ingredients with β-cyclodextrin displayed better solubility than the active ingredients themselves. The products obtained after freeze-drying of a solution of these mixtures yielded increased solubility. This can be explained either by the hydrophilic nature of the freeze-dried products and their amorphous character, or by the existence in the freeze-dried mixture of a varying proportion of preformed inclusion compound.

Solubility diagram and stability constant
Higuchi's [58] solubility analysis method was applied by different authors to various active ingredients in the presence of cyclodextrins. Uekama, for example, studied digitoxin [59], digoxin [60], eighteen steroid hormones

[61], proscillaridin [45], spironolactone [62], clofibrate [21], flurbiprofen [63], propylparaben [64], prostaglandins E_1 [53] and F_{2_α} [27]. This method was also applied by Møllgaard Andersen and Bundgaard to hydrocortisone [34] and to spironolactone [68].

If the solubility increases linearly with cyclodextrin concentration, the curve is said to be of Higuchi's type A_L, and corresponds to the formation of an inclusion compound with the stoichiometry of 1/1. The curves are of Higuchi's type B_S if, after a linear rise, a plateau is observed, followed by a decrease corresponding to the precipitation of a microcrystalline inclusion compound with a different stoichiometry.

The plotting of these diagrams serves to calculate an apparent stability constant from the straight part of the curves. This constant reflects the correct adjustment of the guest molecule inside the cavity of the host molecule. Hence, for example, the stability constants calculated by Seo *et al.* [62] for the inclusion compound of spironolactone with α-, β- and γ-cyclodextrins are 960, 27500 and 7600 M^{-1} respectively. As a rule, steroids display better interaction with β- or γ-cyclodextrins, as α-cyclodextrin is much too small to allow inclusion [61].

Dissolution of inclusion compounds
Solubility diagrams remain too theoretical for practical application, because they are plotted when equilibrium is reached, in other words after four to ten days of agitation. Thus, the analysis of the dissolution kinetics of solid inclusion compounds is often preferable, because this can be used to reveal not only an improvement in solubility, but also the rate of passage into solution. These studies also help to point out the value of using a solid inclusion from the formulation standpoint, rather than the simple physical mixture [38,69], or a freeze-dried or spray-dried product [9,10].

A comparison of the inclusion compounds obtained with different cyclodextrins is interesting. Inclusion compounds with flurbiprofen in β- and γ-cyclodextrins [63] display stability constants of 5100 and 460 M^{-1} respectively, and the crystallinity of the inclusion in γ-cyclodextrin is less pronounced than that of the inclusion in β-cyclodextrin. The results of the dissolution of these substances reveal not only faster dissolution for the γ-cyclodextrin inclusion compound, but also a progressive dissociation of this compound in aqueous medium, rapidly causing precipitation of free flurbiprofen.

For the more convenient study of these dissociation mechanisms, rather than using the dissolution method which consists of dispersing a quantity of test product in the dissolution medium, it is often more interesting to use the rotary disc method. This method offers the advantage of linearizing the dissolution curves when dissolution is uniform, but, on the other hand, if the inclusion compound decomposes in aqueous medium, the released active ingredient reprecipitates, and the curve obtained by the rotary disc method displays a negative curve versus time. Because it offers a particularly clear representation, this method has often been used [45,60-62,68,70,71].

Diffusion through semi-permeable membranes

The foregoing studies help to establish a hypothesis according to which water-soluble inclusion compounds, by dissociation, increase the bioavailability of the active ingredients they contain, a hypothesis which needs to be substantiated. This is why both Szejtli [72] and Uekama [21,62,71,73,74] investigated the possibilities of diffusion of active ingredients or their inclusion compounds through semi-permeable membranes. To do this, they employed systems comprising a cellophane membrane between a donor compartment and an acceptor compartment, each equipped with an agitation system. With the donor and acceptor compartments filled with water, and the test products (active ingredient alone and inclusion compound) added in the solid state to the donor compartment, then the diffusion of the inclusion compound is often not as significant as expected. In some cases, such as fendiline in β-cyclodextrin [72], it is lower than that of the active ingredient alone, and, in other cases, such as that of flurbiprofen in β- and γ-cyclodextrins [71], although it is better than that of the active ingredient alone, it does not agree with the comparative effect of these cyclodextrins on dissolution.

To explain these results Otagiri *et al.* [71] compared them with that obtained by placing the solutions of active ingredient and inclusion compound directly in the donor compartment. In this case, the active ingredient (flurbiprofen) diffused better than the inclusion compound. Diffusion is closely dependent on molecular size, and the inclusion compounds diffuse with greater difficulty than the drug molecules. In addition, diffusion must be related to the stability constant: the higher the constant the less the diffusion (for inclusion compounds, 1/1, of flurbiprofen, $K\beta=5100$ M^{-1} and $K\gamma=460$ M^{-1}).

These studies show that this investigative method is perhaps not a good indication of possible absorption *in vivo*.

Interface transfer

Hoping to develop an experimental model imitating the *in vivo* absorption of inclusion compounds, Uekama *et al.* [64] used an *in vitro* dissolution model $S/L_w/L_o$ (solid phase/aqueous liquid phase/organic liquid phase) [76,77]. The model consists of a rotary disc in an organic phase. With pure substances, a good correlation was observed between the theoretical concentration of product passing from the solid phase to the organic liquid phase and the experimental values. With inclusion compounds, the mechanism was much more complex, and the theoretical calculation of diffusion became problematic. However, the measurement of the concentration in the organic phase always remained a good indication of *in vivo* absorption for active ingredients resorbed by passive diffusion.

In situ *resorption*

In addition to the *in vitro* experimental model, Uekama developed and used an *in situ* experimental model, $S/L_w/in$ *situ* (solid phase/aqueous liquid phase/*in situ*). This model consists of perfusing *in situ* a predetermined length of the small intestine of an anaesthetized rat or rabbit, with an aqueous dissolution liquid of the test product, as its dissolution proceeds, and regularly determining the active ingredient in the blood of the animal. Uekama showed that a good correlation existed between the results of the study of *in vitro* interface transfer and *in situ* absorption.

A study of the same type was carried out by Szejtli and Szente [38] who compared the absorption of indomethacin labelled with ^{14}C, alone or included in β-cyclodextrin, in the small and large intestines of rats. In the case of indomethacin only, 56% was absorbed in the small intestine and 6% in the large intestine. In the case of included indomethacin, absorption was 68 and 66% respectively.

In vivo *investigations — bioavailability and pharmacokinetics*
Whatever the value of the foregoing techniques, they can only offer firm hope of an improvement in bioavailability, and this must be verified in animals and in humans.

Oral administration
The inclusion of an active ingredient in a cyclodextrin may reduce its bitterness [44,78], and, more interestingly, any harmful side-effects, such as the destruction of the stomach mucous membranes by certain non-steroid anti-inflammatory substances. This is what happens with phenylbutazone included in β-cyclodextrin, but is not observed with indomethacin or flufenamic acid [79]. The disappearance of the irritation of pirprofen on the mucous membrane of the throat is reduced by inclusion in β-cyclodextrin [80].

Concerning bioavailability, an improvement is usually observed if the inclusion of an active ingredient has already improved its dissolution. Not only is the blood concentration higher, with its peak occurring sooner, but the area under the curve (plasma concentration/time) is also larger. These results can be obtained, for example, after the oral administration of inclusion compounds of digoxin/γ-cyclodextrin in the dog [59,60], spirono-lactone/β- or γ-cyclodextrin in the dog [62], phenytoin/β-cyclodextrin in the dog [65], flurbiprofen/β- or γ-cyclodextrin in the rabbit [71], acetohexamide/β-cyclodextrin in the rabbit [74], diazepam/γ-cyclodextrin in the rabbit [75], ketoprofen/β-cyclodextrin in the dog [8], ketoprofen, ibuprofen or flufena-mic acid/β-cyclodextrin in the rabbit [8], indomethacin/β-cyclodextrin in the rat [38], but no favourable effect is observed in the rabbit [8], and allobar-bital, amobarbital, barbital, pentobarbital or phenobarbital/β-cyclodextrin in the rabbit [81].

A similar result is obtained by the oral administration in humans of the inclusion compounds salicylic acid/β-cyclodextrin [82] or prednisolone/β-cyclodextrin [73]. These studies also reveal the value of the oral administra-tion of freeze-dried drugs [65,83]. In some cases, the improvement in bioavailability caused by inclusion is such that a reduction in the dose administered can be considered. This applies in particular to the inclusion digoxin/γ-cyclodextrin (1/4) [59,60].

It may sometimes be advantageous to administer an additive at the same time as the inclusion, to imporive its *in vivo* effectiveness. This applies in particular to cinnarizine, whose inclusion in β-cyclodextrin increases its solubility at pH 3.0 to 6.8, but does not change its bioavailability. Accordingly, the stomach pH must be changed to produce better dissolution, and this is done by the simultaneous administration of $NaHCO_3$ [84]. For the same product, the administration of a competing agent, such as DL-phenylalanine, also proves to be interesting. After oral administration, the dissociation of the inclusion cinnarizine/β-cyclodextrin is facilitated by the presence of phenylalanine, which tends to supplant the cinnarizine in the cyclodextrin, causing the absorption of cinnarizine, now in the molecular state, to occur more rapidly [85].

Improved bioavailability should normally be reflected by an increase in therapeutic effect. This was observed by Koizumi, who investigated five barbiturates (phenobarbital, pentobarbital, amobarbital, allobarbital and barbital) [86]. Their effective dose was actually reduced to varying degrees by inclusion in β-cyclodextrin. In addition, with the exception of barbital, the latent time before the induction of sleep was generally shortened, while the duration of sleep was prolonged [86].

Szejtli also observed therapeutic improvements by the administration of vitamin D_3 to rats [28,29,87]. Increases in urinary volume in the rat were observed by the administration of spironolactone included in γ-cyclodextrin, greater than those caused by spironolactone alone [88].

Rectal administration
The rectal administration of suppositories containing active ingredients, alone or in cyclodextrin inclusions, is often reflected by greater bioavailability [71,74,89]. In actual fact, it appears that the type of excipient has a significant effect on the bioavailability of the active ingredient itself or of the inclusion compound [90]. This was observed with phenobarbital included in β-cyclodextrin, combined with Witepsol 55 or with Macrogol. In this case, it should be noted that the cyclodextrin tended to delay the absorption of phenobarbital in the rectum, so that the higher blood concentrations with the inclusion compound can essentially be attributed to a faster release of this compound (hydrophilic) than of the phenobarbital, based on the excipients employed.

Cutaneous administration
Otagiri and Uekama [91,92] investigated the release of betamethasone and the percutaneous absorption of beclomethasone dipropionate included in β- and/or γ-cyclodextrins, using hydrophilic bases. On the whole, the release of the active ingredients, measured through an artificial double-layer membrane or a cellophane membrane, was increased by inclusion. Moreover, in the case of the beclomethasone dipropionate included in γ-cyclodextrin, an increase in the vasoconstrictor effect of the product was observed, which appears to reflect an improvement in percutaneous absorption [92].

Ocular administration
Very few tests have yet been conducted on this method of administration. However, it is worthwhile noting the possibility of reducing local irritation caused by flurbiprofen, when the latter is included in β-cyclodextrin [93]. It also appears that the inclusion of sodium sulfacetamide in β-cyclodextrin improves its release from an ophthalmic ointment [94].

Parenteral administration
While the non-toxicity of cyclodextrins by oral administration appears to be highly probable [95], this cannot be said of parenteral administration. Tests have nevertheless been conducted by this method in animals.

Nagai *et al.* [96] administered hexobarbital in the presence of α-, β- and γ-cyclodextrins in mice and rats by intravenous and intraperitoneal administration. A significant change in the pharmacokinetics of the product resulted from the presence of cyclodextrins. Ten and twenty minutes after intravenous administration, the following effects were observed in comparison with hexobarbital alone: higher blood and kidney concentrations, lower brain and liver concentrations, shorter sleeping time and a prolonged latent period before induction of sleep.

CONCLUSIONS

Cyclodextrins display high inclusion capacity for non-hydrophilic molecules. The inclusion compounds thus formed should normally be extremely valuable in pharmaceutical technology, because it has already been proved that they significantly enhance the storage of many products in the solid state and sometimes in liquid medium. Their greatest value is undoubtedly the possibility of substantially improving the bioavailability of products that are orally administered. There use is likely to spread considerably after the prolonged toxicity investigations have been completed.

REFERENCES

[1] A. Villiers, *C. R. Acad. Sci.*, **111**, 536 (1891).
[2] F. Schardinger and Z. Unters, *Nahrungs. Genussmittel Gebrauchsgegenstände*, **6**, 865 (1903).
[3] F. Schardinger, *Wien Klin. Wochenschr.*, **17**, 207 (1904).
[4] F. Schardinger, *Zentr. Bakteriol. Parasitenk Infektionskr.*, **11**, **29**, 188 (1904).
[5] W. Saenger, *Angew. Chem. Int.*, Ed. Engl., **19**, 344 (1980).
[6] M. Kurozumi, N. Nambu and T. Nagai, *Chem. Pharm. Bull.*, **23**, 3062 (1975).
[7] A. Brétillon, Rapport de DEA de Pharmacie Industrielle, Université de Paris-Sud, 1983.
[8] N. Nambu, M. Shimoda, Y. Takahashi, H. Ueda and T. Nagai, *Chem. Pharm. Bull.*, **26**, 2952 (1978).
[9] M. Kata and A. Antal, *Pharmazie*, **39**, 856 (1984).

[10] M. Kata and M. Lukacs, *Pharmazie*, **39**, 857 (1984).

[11] K. A. Connors and T. W. Rosanka, *J. Pharm. Sci.*, **69**, 173 (1980).

[12] K. Terada, K. Yamamoto and Y. Nakai, 3rd Int. Conf. on Pharmaceutical Technology, Paris, 31 May/2 June 1983, Vol. V, 246.

[13] J. Szejtli and E. Bolla, *Stärke*, **33**, 387 (1981).

[14] D. Duchêne, B. Debruères and C. Vaution, *STP Pharma*, **1**, 37 (1985).

[15] D. Duchêne, C. Vaution and F. Glomot, *STP Pharma*, **1**, 323 (1985).

[16] J. Szejtli, L. Szente and E. Banky-Elöd, *Acta Chim. Acad. Sci. Hung.*, **101**, 27 (1979).

[17] J. Szejtli, L. Szente, T. Zilahy, G. Nagy, M. Gialne Fuzy and J. Haranji, *Hung. Teljes*, HU 24 895, 28 April 1983.

[18] J. Szejtli, L. Szente and I. Apostol, *Hung. Teljes*, HU 22 456, 28 May 1982.

[19] K. Szente, I. Apostol and J. Szejtli, *Pharmazie*, **39**, 697 (1985).

[20] M. Gialne Fuzy, L. Szente, J. Szejtli and J. Haranji, *Pharmazie*, **39**, 558 (1984).

[21] K. Uekama, K. Oh, M. Otagiri, H. Seo and M. Tsuruoka, *Pharm. Acta Helv.*, **58**, 338 (1983).

[22] K. Uekama, F. Hirayama, K. Esaki and M. Inoue, *Chem. Pharm. Bull.*, **27**, 76 (1979).

[23] K. Uekama, S. Narisawa, F. Hirayama, M. Otagiri, K. Kawano, T. Ohtani and H. Ogino, *Int. J. Pharm.*, **13**, 253 (1983).

[24] Y. Nakai, K. Yamamoto, K. Terada and K. Akimoto, *Chem. Pharm. Bull.*, **32**, 685 (1984).

[25] K. Uekama, K. Oh, T. Irie, M. Otagiri, Y. Nishimiya and T. Nara, *Int. J. Pharm.*, **25**, 339 (1985).

[26] F. Møllgaard Andersen and H. Bundgaard, *Int. J. Pharm.*, **19**, 189 (1984).

[27] K. Uekama, F. Hirayama, A. Fujise, M. Otagiri, K. Inaba and H. Saito, *J. Pharm. Sci.*, **73**, 382 (1984).

[28] J. Szejtli and E. Bollan, *Stärke*, **32**, 386 (1980).

[29] J. Szejtli, E. Bolla-Pusztai, P. Szabo and T. Ferenczy, *Pharmazie*, **35**, 779 (1980).

[30] A. Shima and H. Ikura, *Japan Kokai*, JP 77, 130 904, 2 November 1977.

[31] Kyoshin Co. Ltd, *Japan Kokai*, JP 57, 117 671, 1 November 1982.

[32] Y. Yonezawa, S. Maruyama and K. Takagi, *Agric. Biol. Chem.*, **45**, 505 (1981).

[33] J. Szejtli, E. Bolla-Pusztai and M. Kajatar, *Pharmazie*, **37** 725 (1982).

[34] F. Møllgaard Andersen and H. Bundgaard, *Arch. Pharm. Chem.*, *Sci. Ed.*, **11**, 66 (1983).

[35] F. Møllgaard Andersen and H. Bundgaard, *Int. J. Pharm.*, **20**, 155 (1984).

[36] F. Møllgaard Andersen and H. Bundgaard, *Arch. Pharm. Chem.*, *Sci. Ed.*, **10**, 80 (1982).

[37] Y. Nakai, S. Nakajima, K. Yamamoto, K. Terada and T. Konno, *Chem. Pharm. Bull.*, **28**, 1552 (1980).

[38] J. Szejtli and L. Szente, *Pharmazie*, **36**, 694 (1981).
[39] Sumimoto Chemical Co. Ltd., *Japan Kokai*, JP 81, 135 415, 22 October 1981.
[40] Y. Hamada, N. Nambu and T. Nagai, *Chem. Pharm. Bull.*, **23**, 1205 (1975).
[41] T. Nagai, O. Shirakura and N. Nambu, 3rd Int. Conf. on Pharmaceutical Technology, Paris, 31 May/2 June 1983, Vol. V, 253.
[42] S. H. Min, *Yakhah Hoeji*, **16**, 155 (1972).
[43] K. Kyoko and K. Fujimura, *Yakugaku Zasshi*, **92**, 32 (1972).
[44] K. Fujioka, Y. Kurosaky, S. Sato, Te. Noguchi, Ta. Noguchi and Y. Yamahira, *Chem. Pharm. Bull.*, **31**, 2416 (1983).
[45] K. Uekama, T. Fujinaga, M. Otagiri, N. Matsou and Y. Matsuoka, *Acta Pharm. Suec.*, **20**, 287 (1983).
[46] N. Hayasaki, T. Tsutomu, T. Matsumoto and K. Inaba, *Ger. Offen.*, 2 353 797, 9 May 1974.
[47] D. C. Monkhouse, US Pat. 3 952 004, 20 April 1976.
[48] D. C. Monkhouse, US Pat. 3 954 787, 4 May 1976.
[49] M. Hayashi, K. Shuto and Y. Iijima, *Ger. Offen.*, 2 819 447, 9 November 1978.
[50] Ono Pharmaceutical Co. Ltd, *Japan Kokai*, JP 57, 156 460, 27 September 1982.
[51] Ono Pharmaceutical Co. Ltd, *Japan Kokai*, JP 58, 18 357, 2 February 1983.
[52] K. K. Teisan Seiyaku, *Japan Kokai*, JP 59, 10 525, 20 January 1984.
[53] K. Uekama, A. Fujise, F. Hirayama, M. Otagiri and K. Inaba, *Chem. Pharm. Bull.*, **32**, 275 (1984).
[54] P. Hsyu, R. P. Hedge, B. K. Birmingham and C. T. Rhodes, *Drug Develop. Ind. Pharm.*, **10**, 601 (1984).
[55] T. Tokumura, K. Tatsuishi, M. Kayano, Y. Machida and T. Nagai, *Chem. Pharm. Bull.*, **33**, 2079 (1985).
[56] O. I. Corrigan and C. T. Stanley, *Pharm. Acta Helv.*, **56**, 204 (1981).
[57] O. I. Corrigan and C. T. Stanley, *J. Pharm. Pharmacol.*, **34**, 621 (1982).
[58] T. Higuchi and J. L. Lach, *J. Am. Pharm. Assoc., Sci. Ed.*, **43**, 349 (1954).
[59] K. Uekama, T. Fujinaga, F. Hirayama, M. Otagiri, H. Seo and M. Tsuruoka, 1st Int. Symposium on Cyclodextrins, Budapest, 1981, 399.
[60] K. Uekama, T. Fujinaga, F. Hirayama, M. Otagiri, M. Yamasaki, H. Seo, T. Hashimoto and M. Tsuruoka, *J. Pharm. Sci.*, **72**, 1338 (1983).
[61] K. Uekama, T. Fujinaga, F. Hirayama, M. Otagiri and M. Yamasaki, *Int. J. Pharm.*, **10**, 1 (1982).
[62] H. Seo, M. Tsuruoka, T. Hashimoto, T. Fujinaga, M. Otagiri and K. Uekama, *Chem. Pharm. Bull.*, **31**, 286 (1983).
[63] M. Otagiri, T. Imai, F. Hirayama and K. Uekama, *Acta Pharm. Suec.*, **20**, 11 (1983).
[64] K. Uekama, Y. Uemura, T. Irie and M. Otagiri, *Chem. Pharm. Bull.*, **31**, 3637 (1983).

[65] M. Tsuruoka, T. Hashimoto, H. Seo, S. Ichimasa, O. Ueno, T. Fujinaga, M. Otagiri and K. Uekama, *Yakugaku Zasshi*, **101**, 360 (1981).

[66] K. Koizumi, J. Tatsumi, M. Ohae, H. Kumagai and T. Hayata, *Yakugaku Zasshi*, **89**, 1594 (1969).

[67] K. Fujimura and K. Koizumi, *Yakugaku Zasshi*, **92**, 32 (1972).

[68] F. Møllgaard Andersen and H. Bundgaard, *Arch. Pharm. Chem., Sci. Ed.*, **11**, 7 (1983).

[69] J. Szejtli, E. Bolla-Pusztai, M. Tardy-Lengyel, P. Szabb and T. Ferenczy, *Pharmazie*, **38**, 189 (1983).

[70] K. Uekama, Y. Ikeda, F. Hirayama, M. Otagiri and M. Shibata, *Yakigaku Zasshi*, **100**, 994 (1980).

[71] M. Otagiri, T. Imai, N. Matsuo and K. Uekama, *Acta Pharm. Suec.*, **20**, 1 (1983).

[72] A. Stadler-Szöke, M. Vikmon and J. Szejtli, *J. Incl. Phenom.*, **3**, 71 (1985).

[73] K. Uekama, M. Otagiri, Y. Uemura, T. Fujinaga, K. Arimori, N. Matsuo, K. Tasaki and A. Sugii, *Pharm. Dyn.*, **6**, 124 (1983).

[74] K. Uekama, N. Matsuo, F. Hirayama, H. Ichibagase, K. Arimori, K. Tsubaki and K. S. Atake, *Yakugaku Zasshi*, **100**, 903 (1980).

[75] K. Uekama, S. Narisawa, F. Hirayama and M. Otagiri, *Int. J. Pharm.*, **16**, 327 (1983).

[76] K. Uekama, J. Fujisaki and F. Hirayama, *Yakugaku Zasshi*, **100**, 1087 (1980).

[77] K. Uekama, Y. Uemura, F. Hirayama and M. Otagiri, *Chem. Pharm. Bull.*, **31**, 3284 (1983).

[78] F. Møllgaard Andersen, H. Bundgaard and H. B. Mengel, *Int. J. Pharm.*, **21**, 51 (1984).

[79] N. Nambu, K. Kikuchi, T. Kikuchi, Y. Takahashi, H. Ueda and T. Nagai, *Chem. Pharm. Bull.*, **26**, 3609 (1978).

[80] T. Hibi, M. Tatsumi, M. Hanabusa, R. Higuchi, T. Imai, M. Otagiri and K. Uekama, *Yakigaku Zasshi*, **104**, 990 (1985).

[81] K. Koizumi and Y. Kidera, *Yakugaku Zasshi*, **97**, 705 (1977).

[82] K. H. Frömming and I. Weyermann, *Arzneim, Forsch (Drug Res.)*, **23**, 424 (1973).

[83] H. Sekikawa, N. Fukuda, M. Takada, K. Ohtani, T. Arita and M. Nakano, *Chem. Pharm. Bull.*, **31**, 1350 (1983).

[84] T. Tokumura, Y. Tsushima, K. Tatsuishi, M. Kayano, Y. Machida and T. Nagai, *Chem. Pharm. Bull.*, **33**, 2962 (1985).

[85] T. Tokumura, Y. Tsushima, M. Kayano, Y. Machida and T. Nagai, *J. Pharm. Sci.*, **74**, 496 (1985).

[86] K. Koizumi, H. Miki and Y. Kubota, *Chem. Pharm. Bull.*, **28**, 319 (1980).

[87] A. Fonagy, A. Gerloczy, P. Kerestes and J. Szejtli, 1st Int. Symposium on Cyclodextrins, Budapest, 1981, 409.

[88] B. Debruères, A. Brétillon and D. Duchêne, *Proc. Int. Symp. Control Rel. Bioact-Mater.*, **12**, 118 (1985).

[89] A. Stadler-Szöke and J. Szejtli, 1st Int. Symposium on Cyclodextrins, Budapest, 1981, 377.

[90] R. Iwaoku, K. Armori, M. Nakano and K. Uekama, *Chem. Pharm. Bull.*, **30**, 1416 (1982).

[91] M. Otagiri, T. Fujinaga, A. Sakai and K. Uekama, *Chem. Pharm. Bull.*, **32**, 2401 (1984).

[92] K. Uekama, M. Otagiri, A. Sakai, T. Irie, N. Matsuo and Y. Matsuoka, *J. Pharm. Pharmacol.*, **37**, 532 (1985).

[93] K. Masuda, A. Ito, T. Ikari, A. Terashima and T. Matsuyama, *Yakugaku Zasshi*, **104**, 1075 (1984).

[94] N. Shankland and J. R. Johnson, *J. Pharm. Pharmacol.*, **36**, suppl. 21P (1984).

[95] J. Szejtli, *J. Incl. Phenom.*, **2**, 487 (1984).

[96] T. Nagai, O. Shirakuba and N. Nambu, 3rd Int. Conf. on Pharmaceutical Technology, Paris, 31 May/2 June 1983, Vol. V, 263.

2

Stabilization of local anaesthetics in liposomes

M. J. Habib and **J. A. Rogers**
Faculty of Pharmacy and Pharmaceutical Sciences, University of Alberta, Edmonton, Alberta, Canada T6G 2N8

SUMMARY

The first-order hydrolysis rate constants of local anaesthetic drugs have been measured in aqueous buffer solution, k_B, and in liposomes, k_{obs}, at pH 12.2 and 30°C. Also, the fraction of drug associated with the lipid phase, f_L, and the partition coefficient between the aqueous and lipid phase, K_B^L, were determined. The stability of benzocaine was measured in several liposome compositions, and as a function of benzocaine concentration, phospholipid concentration and ionic strength of the medium. Values of the rate constant in the lipid phase, k_L were estimated from a simple kinetic model and predictions of the relative contributions of k_L and k_B to k_{obs} were made. Different methods of liposome preparation, and the stabilities of local anaesthetics in liposomal and micellar systems were compared.

INTRODUCTION

Liposomes are colloidal dispersions of lipid molecules arranged as bimolecular leaflets in an approximately spherical shape and enclosing compartments of aqueous medium. These easily prepared formulations have created considerable interest in studies of drug–membrane interactions [1] and as drug delivery systems [2]. Recently, and interesting potential application of liposomes to stabilize drugs has been given some attention [3–6]. These attempts have been mainly aimed at incorporating drug into phospholipid bilayers by equilibrium partitioning with the expectation that the hydrocarbon environment of the bilayer offers protection against catalytic hydrolysis in a manner similar to that found in micellar systems [7–9].

Depending on the composition of the liposomes and the chemical nature of the solute, increases in stability have ranged from 0% (e.g. cyclocytidine [5]) to about 90% for a trimethylammonium halide [6]. These results indicate that the important factors involved in the stabilization of esters or amides in liposomes are the depth of the reactive centre of the solute molecule in the phospholipid bilayer membrane [6] and the fraction of the total drug associated [5] with or partitioned [3] in the liposomes. There is also evidence, however, that drug bound to sites in the bilayers may also give rise to improved stability [10] whereas ester adsorbed or bound to the liposome surfaces can accelerate its loss in comparison to its concentration in aqueous buffer solution [11].

Local anaesthetic drugs are esters whose hydrolysis kinetics have been studied in aqueous solution [12, 13] and micelles [14–16]. Procaine has also been stabilized in neutral, fluid liposomes [3] and in lyotropic smectic mesophases [17]. A study of a series of these agents in liposome systems under various conditions offers a convenient means of determining the importance of the role of partitioning on stability in this type of formulation.

MATERIALS

The lipids used as received in this study were supplied by Sigma Chemical Co., St. Louis, Missouri and included: L-α-dimyristoylphosphatidylcholine, 98% (DMPC), L-α-dipalmitoylphosphatidylcholine, 99% (DPPC), L-α-phosphatidylcholine, type V-E from egg yolk (EPC), sphingomyelin from bovine brain (SPHING), phosphatidylserine from bovine brain, 98% (PS), and cholesterol, 99% (CHOL). Local anaesthetics included benzocaine, USP (J. T. Baker Chemical Co.), procaine hydrochloride, USP (Allen & Hanbury), tetracaine hydrochloride (Sigma Chemical Co.), methyl p-amino-benzoate, 97%, n-propyl p-aminobenzoate, 99%, and n-butyl p-aminobenzoate, 97% (Pfaltz & Bauer). Indomethacin (Sigma Chemical Co.) was also studied for comparison. The degradation products, p-aminobenzoic acid (Allen & Hanbury) and 4-(butylamino) benzoic acid, 98% (Aldrich Chemical Co.) were required in the analytical procedure. All other chemicals and solvents were reagent grade and water was glass-distilled.

METHODS

Aqueous buffer solutions used in these studies had the following compositions: $0.059M$ $KH_2PO_4 + 0.007M$ Na_2HPO_4 (pH 6.0), $0.013M$ $KH_2PO_4 + 0.054M$ Na_2HPO_4 (pH 7.4), $0.06M$ boric acid $+ 0.14M$ Na_2CO_3 (pH 10.0), and $0.045M$ NaOH (pH 12.2). The ionic strength was adjusted with NaCl usually to 0.15 and checked using an osmometer (Model 3D, Advanced osmometer, Advanced Instruments, Mass.).

Liposome preparation

A stock multilamellar liposome preparation was made as previously described [18]. Briefly, a film of phospholipid (57 micromoles) was formed on the inside wall of a 1 litre round-bottom flask by first dissolving the

phospholipid and chloroform then removing the solvent by rotary evaporation at 40°. It was subsequently flushed with N_2 gas then placed in a
vacuum oven at 40° to dry over P_2O_5 for 12–14 h to remove the last traces of
solvent. Liposomes were formed by adding 10 ml of aqueous buffer solution
warmed to at least 10° above the phase transition temperature of the
phospholipid then vortex-mixed for 10 min. Drugs were incorporated into
liposomes by mixing equal volumes of liposomes and aqueous buffer
solution of drug and thoroughly mixing. Some experiments were conducted
in which the drug was initially incorporated in liposomes via the organic
phase. Thus, procaine was added along with the phospholipid (5 litre
micromoles) to chloroform and a film produced in the usual manner.
Liposomes were then formed after the addition of aqueous buffer solution
(20 ml) as before.

Kinetic studies and analysis

The stabilities of the local anaesthetics were determined in aqueous buffer
solution and in liposomes at pH 12.2 and 30°. Similar conditions have been
used by others [14] in stability studies of benzocaine in micellar solutions
because of the convenient rate of hydrolysis under these conditions and the
constancy of the OH^- concentration during the hydrolysis reactions. The
liposome preparation was divided into 2 ml quantities, placed in 25 ml
stoppered volumetric flasks, then maintained at constant temperature in a
shaking water-bath (Dubnoff metabolic shaker, Precision Scientific Co.). A
test sample was diluted to volume with isopropyl alcohol after a designated
time interval resulting in a clear solution, then assayed spectrophotometri-
cally at λ_{max} (uv/vis Model 25 spectrophotometer, Beckman Instruments,
Inc. CA).

Since the degradation product of the local anaesthetics caused interference in the analysis, the total absorbance (A_λ) in the system is given by

$$A_\lambda = \varepsilon C + \varepsilon_1 C_1 \tag{1}$$

where C and C_1 are the concentrations of reactants and degradation
products, respectively, and ε and ε_1 are their respective apparent molar
absorptivities at λ_{max}. The fraction of drug remaining is determined at any
given time from Eqn. (2):

$$C/C_0 = \frac{A_\lambda/C_0 - \varepsilon_1}{\Delta\varepsilon} \tag{2}$$

where C_0 is the initial concentration of drug, and C is its concentration at
time, t, and $\Delta\varepsilon = \varepsilon - \varepsilon_1$. The values of ε and ε_1 at their respective λ_{max} are
given in Table 1.

The fraction of drug associated with the phospholipid phase (f_L) at the
beginning of the kinetic studies was determined from the difference between
the total amount of drug in the liposomal suspension (D_T) and the residual

Table 1 — Structures and spectral characteristics of local anaesthetics and their degradation products

Local anaesthetic	Structure[a]	λ(nm)	Molar absorptivity
Benzocaine	X=C$_3$H$_7$, Y=H	291	21 552
Procaine	X=C$_2$H$_4$−N$\diagup^{C_2H_5}_{\diagdown C_2H_5}$ Y=H	293	22 747
Tetracaine	X=C$_2$H$_4$−N$\diagup^{CH_3}_{\diagdown CH_3}$ Y=C$_4$H$_9$	309	29 552
Methyl p-amino benzoate	X=CH$_3$, Y=H	294	18 934
n-Propyl p-amino benzoate	X=C$_3$H$_7$, Y=H	294	19 235
n-Butyl p-amino benzoate	X=C$_4$H$_9$, Y=H	294	19 156
p-Aminobenzoic acid	X=H, Y=H	291	5 721
		293	4 946
		294	4 944
p-Butylamino- benzoic acid	X=H, Y=C$_4$H$_9$	309	5 437

[a]General structure: Y−HN−⟨benzene ring⟩−CO−O−X

amount of drug in the supernatant (D_B) after centrifugation (135 000 xg, 30 min, 30°; L8-55 ultracentrifuge, Beckman Instruments Inc. California) divided by D_T.

Partition coefficients in liposomes
Liposomes, which were freshly prepared in aqueous buffer at a lower pH to minimize degradation but maintaining the drug in a completely unionized state, were equilibrated at 30° for 30 min then centrifuged as before at the same temperature at 135 000 xg for 30 min. Subsequently the supernatant was carefully withdrawn by Pasteur pipette, diluted with isopropyl alcohol and analysed spctrophotometrically. Concentrations of drug in the supernatants, C_B, were determined from a calibration curve and the residual amounts in the phospholipid phase were calculated from the mass balance. The molal partition coefficients, K_B^L, were determined from Eqn. (3):

$$K_B^L = \frac{(C_T - C_B)w_1}{C_B \cdot w_2} \tag{3}$$

where C_T is the total concentration of drug (mg/ml) in the system, w_1 and w_2 are the weights of the aqueous and phospholipid phases, respectively.

All kinetic and partition coefficient experiments were performed at least in triplicate and the results averaged.

RESULTS

The hydrolysis of the local anaesthetics in aqueous buffer solution or in liposome preparations obeyed apparent first-order kinetics for at least three half-lives as shown in Fig. 1 and is given by Eqn. (4):

$$C/C_0 = e^{-kt} \tag{4}$$

where C_0 and C are the molar concentrations of drug initially and at time t, respectively, and k is the pseudo first-order hydrolysis rate constant. For hydrolysis in aqueous buffer solution $k = k_B$ and in liposome systems $k = k_{obs}$. Hydrolysis in the lipid phase (k_L) and in the external aqueous phase of liposomes (k_b) was taken to obey Eqn. (4) and that $k_b = k_B$ [5]. Thus,

$$k_{obs} = k_L f_L + k_B f_B \tag{5}$$

where f_L and f_B are the fraction of drug in the lipid and aqueous phases, respectively.

Determination of the relative improvement in the stabilities of liposomes of various compositions was made from the results of k_{obs} and k_B expressed as

$$\% \text{ increase in stability} = \frac{k_B - k_{obs}}{k_B} \times 100 \tag{6}$$

Table 2 indicates a significant variation in the stabilization of benzocaine (a fourfold change) by selecting different phospholipids or phospholipid: cholesterol combinations. Neutral liposomes of phosphatidylcholines, which exist in a fluid liquid crystalline state (EPC, DMPC) at the temperature of the experiment (30°), protects benzocaine against hydrolysis to the extent of 35–40%. In contrast, DPPC is in a more rigid gel state at this temperature and the stability is increased by only 23%.

Sphingomyelin liposomes, although in a fluid state, allow benzocaine to be stabilized only to the extent of 22%. On the other hand, negatively-charged liposomes of PS yield the greatest protection against hydrolysis under the present conditions. The addition of CHOL to DMPC liposomes causes k_{obs} to increase and at a 1:1 mole ratio only a 12% increase in the stability of benzocaine was obtained. Thus, the addition of 50% CHOL to the liposome composition results in about a three-fold decrease in effectiveness of the phospholipid (DMPC) liposomes to stabilize benzocaine.

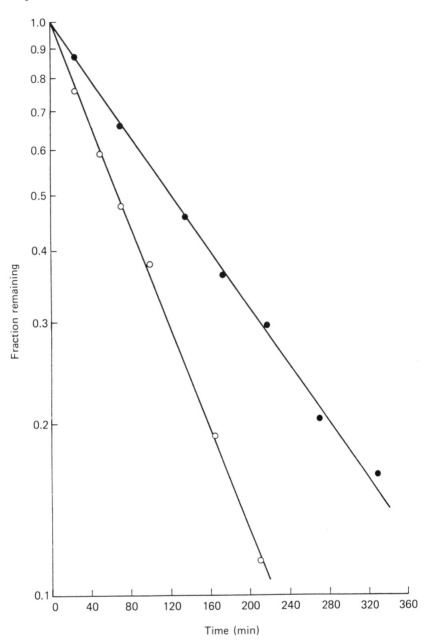

Fig. 1 — First-order hydrolysis kinetics of benzocaine in aqueous buffer solution ○, and in liposomes ●, at pH 12.2 (0.045M NaOH) and 30°C. The initial benzocaine concentration was 0.76 mM and the phospholipid (DMPC) concentration was 5.8 mM.

Table 2 — The stabilization of benzocaine in liposomes of various compositions at pH 12.2 and 30°C[a]

Liposome composition[b]	% Increase in stability[c]
PS	47
EPC	39
DMPC	34
DPPC	23
SPHING	22
DMPC:CHOL (3:1)	25
DMPC:CHOL (1:1)	12

[a]The initial benzocaine concentration was 0.76 mM; the total lipid concentration was 2.9 mM.
[b]See text for definition of abbreviations; mole ratios are shown in parentheses.
[c]Using Eqn. (6).

Studies were conducted to determine whether variation of the content of benzocaine in liposomes or the osmolarity of the aqueous medium produced significant change in the kinetics of degradation. The results in Fig. 2 show a parallel decrease in k_{obs} with increasing benzocaine concentra-

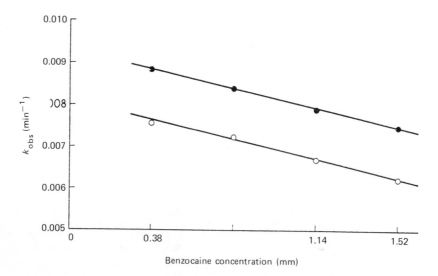

Fig. 2 — Effect of the benzocaine concentration on the hydrolysis rate constant (k_{obs}) in liposomes at pH 12.2 and 30°C. DMPC, ○; DPPC, ●.

tion in liposomes of DMPC or DPPC. However, a fourfold increase in benzocaine concentration resulted in only a 15% decrease in k_{obs}. Similarly, ionic strengths of the aqueous medium ranging from 0.05 to 0.25 had little effect on k_{obs} (Table 3) even though the liposomes exist in various swelling

Table 3 – Hydrolysis rate constants of benzocaine in DMPC liposomes (k_{obs}) as a function of the ionic strength of the medium at pH 12.2 and 30°C[a]

Ionic strength	$10^3 k_{obs}$ (SD)
0.046	7.3 (0.20)
0.060	7.2 (0.19)
0.100	6.9 (0.13)
0.154 (isotonic)	6.8(0.09)
0.250	6.8(0.11)

[a]The initial benzocaine concentration was 0.76 mM; the DMPC concentration was 2.9 mM.

states under these conditions [19].

The variation of k_{obs} of benzocaine, procaine and tetracaine in DMPC or DPPC liposomes as a function of the phospholipid concentration over the range 1.4–28.7 mM is illustrated in Fig. 3. Each curve is characterized by an initial rapid decrease in k_{obs} followed by a more gradual lowering of k_{obs} as the phospholipid is further increased. The steepness of the slopes in the initial stages corresponding to DMPC liposomes is in the order benzocaine > procaine > tetracaine which is also the same order as their partition coefficients whereas the latter segments of the curves are approximately parallel. In contrast, the curve corresponding to benzocaine in DPPC liposomes exhibits a more gradual change indicating that k_{obs} is much less influenced by the amount of lipid when the liposomes exist in the gel state. However, it is significant to observe that in fluid DMPC liposomes the relative increase in stability of benzocaine or procaine parallels the increase in f_L (Table 4) whereas approximately a four-fold increase in the stability of tetracaine is obtained by a 40% increase in f_L at the higher DMPC concentration.

Incorporation of local anaesthetics into liposomes for the purpose of stabilization appears also to be pH dependent. Thus, the procaine stability data in Table 5 indicates that only undissociated procaine is able to accumulate in the lipid phase when introduced via the aqueous phase because at pH 7.4, at which procaine is 96% ionized ($pK_a = 8.8$), only 4% increase in stability was obtained. However, most of the increase in the stability of procaine at pH 12.2 is recoverable of pH 7.4 if the drug is incorporated in liposomes via the organic phase during preparation.

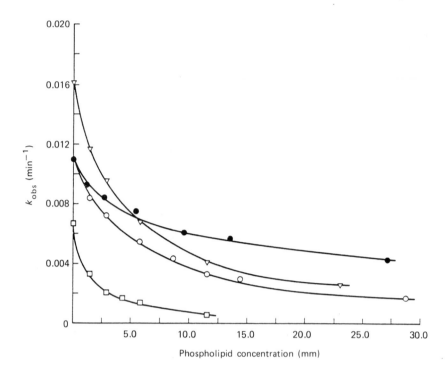

Fig. 3 — Effect of phospholipid concentration on the hydrolysis rate constant (k_{obs}) of local anaesthetics in liposomes at pH 12.2 and 30°C. The initial drug concentration was 0.76 mM. Benzocaine (DMPC), O; (DPPC), ●; procaine (DMPC), ∇; tetracaine (DMPC), □.

Table 4 — Relationship between the initial fraction in the lipid phase (f_L) and the relative stability (k_{obs}/k_B) of local anaesthetics in liposomes as a function of the phospholipid (DMPC) concentration[a]

Local anaesthetic[b]	DMPC Conc. (mM)	f_L	k_{obs}/k_B
Benzocaine	2.9	0.28	0.66
	11.5	0.63	0.31
Procaine	2.9	0.26	0.60
	11.5	0.64	0.25
Tetracaine	2.9	0.63	0.31
	11.5	0.88	0.08

[a]Experiments were conducted at pH 12.2 and 30°C.
[b]Initial concentrations were 0.76 mM.

Table 5 — Effect of the method of incorporation of procaine in liposomes on its stability at 30°C[a]

	% Increase in stability	
Incorporation of procaine	pH 12.2	pH 7.4
Via aqueous phase	41.0	4.0
Via organic phase	43.0	30.0

[a]DMPC concentration = 2.9 mM; procaine conc. = 0.76 mM.

DISCUSSION

The kinetics of benzocaine hydrolysis in liposomes of various compositions differed significantly as shown in Table 2. Thus, association of the drug with the lipid phase appears to be responsible for a lower k_{obs} than k_B. A possible reason for the reduced hydrolysis in liposomes is the reduced reactivity in the lipid phase of that fraction of drug associated with it, in particular that which is partitioned deep in the bilayers. Thus, solutes which have a low k_L and a substantial f_L may be predicted to yield the greatest decrease in k_{obs}. Liposomal compositions which augment either of these parameters should provide stability improvement. The influence of f_L on bezocaine stability is well illustrated from the evidence of k_{obs} under the influence of varying concentrations of benzocaine (Fig. 2), DMPC (Fig. 3 and Table 4) and ionic strength (Table 3). However, the respective contributions of k_L and f_L to k_{obs} are not as obvious in liposomes of different compositions. For example, in liposomes of decreased bilayer fluidity less drug is able to be accommodated but the magnitude of k_L is not necessarily significantly different than in more fluid liposomes. The occurrence of a phase transition from a fluid liquid crystalline state to a more rigid gel-like state is a characteristic of phospholipids and for DMPC [20] the phase transition temperature (T_c) is 23° whereas it is 41° for DPPC [20] and 25°–40° for SPHING [21]. The partition coefficient of solutes in liposomes often exhibits a remarkable decrease upon cooling liposomes below the t_c [22–26] which is believed to be due to the higher energy requirement of accommodation of solute molecules in the rigid gel state of the bilayers [23]. Thus, the increase in stability of benzocaine in DPPC liposomes is lower because less benzocaine associates with these bilayers. In a similar fashion reduced benzocaine accommodation in DMPC:CHOL liposomes, due to the decreased fluidity [1], contributes to its lower observed stability. Reduced binding, partitioning and stability of solutes in fluid liposomal membranes to which CHOL has been added has been previously reported [25–28]. Although there is no direct evidence of the reactivity in PS or SPHING liposomes, differences in permeability to OH^- may be a major contributing factor. In the case of PS liposomes, strong negatively-charged sites at the liposome surfaces repel OH^- and, therefore, catalytic attack of the reactive centres of benzocaine molecules partitioned in the bilayers is reduced. In contrast, the permeability of SPHING bilayers, like other phospholipids, is greater in the region of its T_c [19] and the result is increased OH^- penetration and hydrolytic attack of benzocaine molecules in the bilayers.

The degradation of the local anaesthetics in liposomes may be described by a simple kinetic model as depicted in Scheme 1:

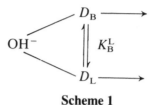

Scheme 1

where D_B and D_L correspond to drug in the aqueous buffer solution and the lipid phase, respectively. The overall rate of hydrolysis is expressed accordingly [14].

$$-(V_B + V_C)\frac{dC}{dt} = k_B V_B C_B + k_L V_L C_L \tag{7}$$

where V_B and V_L are the volumes of the aqueous and lipid phases, respectively, C_B and C_L are the concentrations of drug in each phase, and C refers to the total concentration in the system. V_L was estimated from the density of 1.02 of hydrated lipid [3]. Since $K_B^L = C_L/C_B$, then Eqn. (7) may be expressed as

$$\frac{-d \ln C}{dt} = \frac{k_B - k_L}{1 + K_B^L \dfrac{V_L}{V_B}} + k_L = k_{obs} \tag{8}$$

and following rearrangement gives

$$k_{obs} + \frac{k_{obs}}{K_B^L \dfrac{V_L}{V_B}} = \frac{k_B}{K_B^L \dfrac{V_L}{V_B}} + k_L \tag{9}$$

A plot of this linear relationship yields k_B and k_L from the slope and intercept, respectively, and for benzocaine, procaine, and tetracaine these are shown in Fig. 4. Table 6 compares k_B determined from Eqn. (9) with k_B obtained experimentally. The excellent agreement found supports the validity of Scheme 1 in describing the events occurring during the degradation of these three local anaesthetics. Values of k_L determined from the intercepts were very low (in the order of 10^{-4}–10^{-5} min^{-1}) and were only about 0.5–1.0% of k_B indicating a strong protective capability of liposomes against hydrolysis of local anaesthetics. A comparison of the reactivity in the

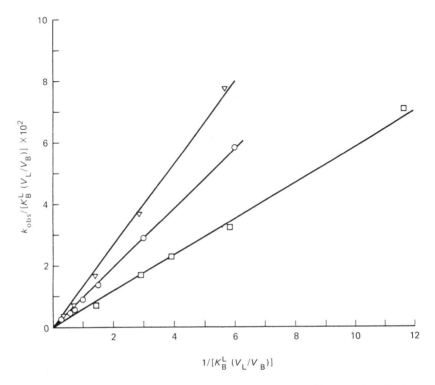

Fig. 4 — Plots of Eqn. (9) for benzocaine, $\bigcirc$; procaine, $\triangledown$; tetracaine, $\square$. A multiplication factor of 10 was applied to both axes for tetracaine.

Table 6 — Comparisons of hydrolysis in aqueous buffer solution (k_B), hydrolysis of associated drug relative to free (k_L/k_B) and contribution of the phospholipid phase to hyrolysis in the liposomal suspension ($k_L f_L/k_{obs}$)

Local Anaesthetic	$k_B(\text{min}^{-1})$ (calc'd)	$k_B(\text{min}^{-1})$ (expt'l)	10^2 k_L/k_B	10^3 $k_L f_L/k_{obs}$
Benzocaine	0.010	0.011	1.2	4.5
Procaine	0.014	0.016	1.0	4.3
Tetracaine	0.006	0.007	0.4	8.4

lipid phase to that in the total liposomal suspension (last column, Table 6) not only emphasizes the impact of a low k_L but also the significance of a higher f_L of tetracaine with respect to the observed increase in its stability.

The stabilization of undissociated drugs such as the local anaesthetics under the present conditions would appear to be strongly influenced by K_B^L. For example, values of K_B^L for benzocaine, procaine, and tetracaine of 169, 180, and 873 correspond to a 34%, 41% and 69% increase in stability, respectively. A test of such correlation is demonstrated in Fig. 5 which also

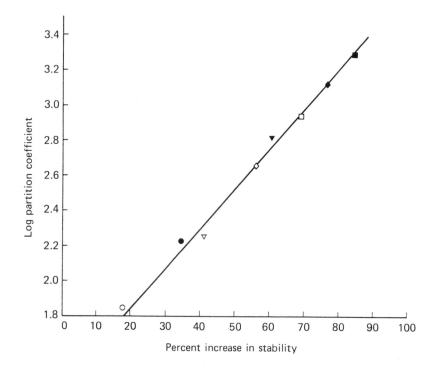

Fig. 5 — Correlation of the partition coefficient (K_B^L) and the observed percent increase in stability of various local anaesthetics and other solutes in DMPC liposomes at pH 12.2 and 30°C. The curve was determined using linear regression analysis ($r = 0.996$). Methyl p-aminobenzoate, ○; benzocaine, ●; procaine, ▽; n-propyl p-amino bonzoate, ▼; tetracaine, □; n-butyl p-aminobenzoate, ■; 2-dimethylaminoethyl p-nitrobenzoate (ref. 4), ◇; indomethacin (ref. 5), ◆.

includes data points for other local anaesthetics and solutes whose stabilities in liposomes have been previously reported [4, 5]. An excellent correlation ($r = 0.996$) was obtained suggesting the possibility of predicting the degree of stabilization of a non-ionic or undissociated drug in a liposome formulation from its liposome K_B^L.

Similarities between micellar and liposome systems have been referred to previously [5]. However, phospholipid bilayers also have properties characteristic of lyotropic smectic mesophases [17, 30]. An indication of which physical state is most predominant in stabilizing drugs is given by a comparison of the stabilization of local anaesthetics in liposomes and surfactant micelles given in Table 7. On a mole per mole basis stabilization in liposomes on average is approximately 50% greater than in micellar systems and this would suggest that the liposomal bilayers in the liquid crystalline state may have some characteristics of a lyotropic smectic mesophase. For example, the hydrolysis reaction rate of procaine hydrochloride in lyotropic liquid crystalline phases of polyoxethylene tridecyl ether was found to be approximately 300-fold slower than in aqueous media [17].

Table 7 — Comparison of the micellar and liposomal stabilization of local anaesthetics

Local anaesthetic	Surfactant[a]	% Increase in stability	
		Micelles (ref.)	Liposomes[b]
Benzocaine	POE 24 monocetyl ether ($\sim$ 4.5 mM)	39.4 [14]	34.0
	C-30 ($\sim$ 12 mM)	58.0 [16]	34.0
	SLS (9.3 mM)	35.6 [16]	34.0
Procaine	PLE (8.3 mM)	50.5 [15]	41.0
	SLS (10 mM)	65.3 [15]	41.0
	CTAB (4 mM)	39.1 [15]	41.0
	N-dodecyl betaine (2mM)	18.3 [15]	41.0
n-Butyl-p-aminobenzoate	POE 24 monocetyl ether ($\sim$ 4.5 mM)	55.7 [14]	84.5

[a] C-30 = Cetyl alcohol polyoxyethylene ethers; SLS = Sodium lauryl sulphate; PLE = Polyoxyethylene lauryl ether; CTAB = Cetyltrimethylammonium bromide.
[b] DMPC concentration = 0.2% (= 2.9 mM).

It appears that ionized drugs may also be stabilized in liposomes but only if they are first incorporated directly into the lipid phase prior to liposome formation. In this case, the mechanisms responsible for decreased reactivity in the lipid phase are probably due to electrostatic complexation with the polar groups of the phospholipid molecules. However, the fraction of total drug which can be stabilized in this manner is limited by the number of available binding sites.

ACKNOWLEDGEMENTS

Financial support from the Medical Research Council of Canada (MA-8659) is gratefully acknowledged. An award of a Canadian Commonwealth Scholarship and an Alberta Heritage Foundation for Medical Research Studentship Research Allowance to M.J.H. is greatly appreciated.

REFERENCES

[1] D. Papahadjopoulos and K. K. Kimelberg, *Prog. Surf. Sci.*, **4**, 1 (1973).

[2] D. Papahadjopoulos, *Ann. N.Y. Acad. Sci.*, **308**, 1, 46 (1978).

[3] T. Yotsuyanagi, T. Hamada, H. Tomida and K. Ikeda, *Acta Pharm. Suec.*, **16**, 271 (1979).

[4] T. Yotsuyanagi, T. Hamada, H. Tomida and K. Ikeda, *Acta Pharm. Suec.*, **16**, 325 (1979).

[5] J. B. D'Silva and R. E. Notari, *J. Pharm Sci.*, **71**, 1394 (1982).

[6] A. A. Fatah and L. M. Leow, *J. Org. Chem.*, **48**, 1886 (1983).

[7] R. B. Dunlop and E. H. Cordes, *J. Phys. Chem.*, **73**, 361 (1963).

[8] A. H. Fendler and L. J. Fendler, in *Catalystsd in Micellar and Macromolecular Systems*, Academic Press, New York, 1975, p. 104.

[9] D. Attwood and A. T. Florence, *Surfactant Systems: Their Chemistry, Pharmacy and Biology*, Chapman & Hall, New York, 1983, p. 739.

[10] M. J. Habib and J. A. Rogers, *45th Int. Congr. Pharm. Sci., Fed. Int. Pharm., Montreal, 1985*, p. 45.

[11] S. K. Pejaver and R. E. Notari, *J. Pharm. Sci.*, **74**, 1167 (1985).

[12] B. Karlen and A. Agren, *Acta Chem. Scand.*, **14**, 197 (1960).

[13] T. Higuchi, A. Havinga and L. W. Busse, *J. Amer. Pharm. Assoc., Sci. Ed.*, **39**, 405 (1950).

[14] G. G. Smith, D. R. Kennedy and J. G. Nairn, *J. Pharm. Sci.*, **63**, 712 (1974).

[15] H. T. Tomida, T. Yotsuyanagi and K. Ikeda, *Chem. Pharm. Bull.*, **26**, 148 (1978).

[16] S. Riegelman, *J. Am. Pharm. Assoc., Sci. Ed.*, **49**, 339 (1960).

[17] K. S. Murthy and E. G. Rippie, *J. Pharm. Sci.*, **59**, 459 (1970).

[18] M. J. Habib and J. A. Rogers, 1st National Meeting, AAPS, Washington, D.C. 1986, Abst. no. 136.

[19] J. de Gier, M. C. Blok, P. W. M. van Dijk, C. Mombers, A. J. Verkley, E. C. M. van der Neut-Kok and L. L. M. van Deenen, *Ann. N.Y. Acad. Sci.*, **308**, 85 (1978).

[20] D. C. Melchior and J. M. Steim, *Ann. Rev. Biophys. Bioeng.*, **5**, 205 (1976).

[21] G. Gregoriadis, C. Kirby, P. Large, A. Meehan and J. Senior, in *Targeting of Drugs*, G. Gregoriadis, J. Senior and A. Trouet (eds), Plenum Press, New York, 1982, p. 155.

[22] Y. Katz and J. M. Diamond, *J. Membr. Biol.*, **17**, 101 (1974).

[23] J. A. Rogers and S. S. Davis, *Biochim. Biophys. Acta*, **598**, 392 (1980).

[24] G. V. Betageri and J. A. Rogers, *Int. J. Pharm.*, in press..

[25] B. J. Forrest and J. Mattari, *Biochem. Biophys. Res. Commun.*, **114**, 1001 (1983).

[26] M. Ahmed, J. S. Burton, J. Hadgraft and I. W. Kellaway, *Biochem. Pharmacol.*, **29**, 236 (1980).

[27] M. J. Conrad and S. J. Singer, *Biochemistry*, **20**, 808 (1981).

[28] R. Ueoka and Y. J. Matsumoto, *J. Org. Chem.*, **49**, 3774 (1984).
[29] M. A. Singer and M. K. Jain, *Can. J. Biochem.*, **58**, 815 (1980).
[30] S. Friberg, *Naturwissenschaften*, **64**, 612 (1977).

3

Processing factors influencing the stability of freeze-dried sodium ethacrynate

R. J. Yarwood†, A. J. Phillips,
Merck, Sharp and Dohme Research Laboratories, Hoddesdon, Herts EN11 9BU, UK, and
J. H. Collett,
Department of Pharmacy, University of Manchester, Manchester M13 9PL, UK

SUMMARY

The transitions observed in differential thermal analysis and electrical conductivity profiles of aqueous sodium ethacrynate systems confirmed their potential to produce different physical forms of drug during freeze drying. The stability of freeze-dried preparations was found to be related to the freezing rate, the concentration of sodium ethacrynate in the pre-lyophilized solution and the fill volume of solution. The stability profiles of the freeze-dried preparations were related to the physical form of the drug and the production of a liquid degradation product.

INTRODUCTION

The freeze-drying process, also referred to as lyophilization, is often used to prepare stable parenteral formulations of drugs that are unstable in aqueous solution. The physical form, chemical stability and dissolution characteristics of these products can be influenced by the conditions under which freeze drying takes place. The poor stability of ethacrynic acid in aqueous solution indicates that commercial preparations should be freeze dried (Edecrin,

† Present address: Wyeth Research (UK) Ltd, Taplow, Berks SL6 0PH, UK.

MSD). Hagerman *et al.* [1] have determined that the stability of the commercial preparation is dependent upon the physical form of the drug obtained. They found that sodium ethacrynate could be freeze dried as the chemically stable crystalline form or as the less stable amorphous form.

In this study an investigation is made of the influence of solution cooling rate, initial concentration of solute and the fill volume on the physical form and stability of freeze-dried sodium ethacrynate. These parameters are characterized by the transitions observed in differential thermal analysis (DTA) and electrical conductivity (EC) profiles and also the solubility of the drug within a system.

MATERIALS AND METHODS
Materials
Ethacrynic acid BP was obtained from Merck, Sharp and Dohme, Hoddes-don, Herts. All other reagents were analytical grade.

Differential thermal analysis — electrical conductivity studies
The system used for these studies was that described by Phillips [2]. Sample solutions (0.5, 2.0 and 4.0% w/w sodium ethacrynate) were prepared in distilled water. Distilled water was used as the reference solution. Equal volumes (3 ml) of sample and reference solutions were used for each determination. Cooling and heating rates were controlled by adjusting the sample holder to be either immersed in liquid nitrogen or held in the cold vapour steam above the surface of the liquid nitrogen.

Freeze-drying studies
Solutions containing known concentrations of sodium ethacrynate were freeze dried in 20 ml vials. The influence of selected freezing rates on the chemical and physical stability of the final preparation was investigated. The studies were programmed using solutions filled into thin, neutral glass, flat-bottomed vials and loosely stoppered with butyl rubber plugs specifically designed for freeze drying. The aqueous solutions of sodium ethacrynate were prepared as described [3] previously and known volumes were filled into the vials. The butyl stoppers were placed loosely in the vials and the contents were frozen using a slow freezing process to −25°C or by fast freezing to −50°C prior to drying in an Edwards Model L10 freeze-drying unit. The dried products were sealed under vacuum. Details of the individual experiments are given below.

Solutions cooled slowly
The loosely stoppered vials containing 2 ml of 2% w/v solution of sodium ethacrynate were frozen slowly to −25°C on the shelves of the freeze drier over a period of 4 h. The drying chamber was then evacuated and the samples dried under vacuum for 48 h until the chamber pressure and product temperature remained constant. The drying chamber was isolated and the vials sealed under vacuum.

Solutions cooled rapidly

The loosely stoppered vials containing 0.5, 1, 2 or 3 ml of 1, 2, 3 or 4% w/v solutions of sodium ethacrynate were loaded randomly on to one of the precooled shelves ($-50°C$) of the freeze-drying unit such that the shelf was fully loaded. The shelves were maintained at $-50°C$ for 4 h. Drying and stoppering was accomplished using the same procedures as described for the slow cooled products.

Moisture content determination

A known weight of sample was dissolved in anhydrous methanol and the total weight present in each sample determined by automatic titration (Methrohm E547/3-20, Roth Scientific Equipment, Farnborough, Hants) with Karl Fischer reagent, the end point being determined amperometrically. Duplicate determinations were made for each sample and the average water content recorded as a w/w percentage.

Storage and stability of freeze-dried sodium ethacrynate

Samples of sodium ethacrynate were stored at 60°C and assayed at selected intervals by the HPLC procedure described previously [4].

Determination of physical form of freeze

Dried sodium ethacrynate

The physical form of the freeze-dried samples was determined by power X-ray diffraction (Model XRD-5, Philips, Cambridge) and by microscopy (W. Watson and Sons Ltd, Barnet, Herts).

RESULTS

DTA and EC studies

The DTA profiles for solutions containing 0.5% w/w of sodium ethacrynate (Fig. 1) show a shallow endotherm starting at $-1.8°C$ and continuing to $-1.5°C$. An additional endotherm was often seen at the end of this shallow endotherm followed by an exotherm and then the liquidus endotherm. The exception to this pattern was the slow cooled–slow heated sample (b) in which small additional endotherms were seen in the middle of the shallow endotherm, there was no apparent liquidus endotherm, and a large exotherm was noted between $-1.5°C$ and 5°C. No thermal events were observed below $-2°C$. For all the 0.5% w/w sodium ethacrynate samples, the EC profile indicated a decrease in resistance starting at $-2°C$ and reaching a miniumum or near minimum at $-1.5°C$. The EC profiles generally showed a two-step decrease in resistance with the exception of the slow cooled–slow heated samples (b) which produced a smooth resistance decrease with time.

The DTA and EC profiles of solutions containing 2% w/w sodium ethacrynate were similar to those obtained for solutions containing 0.5% w/w sodium ethacrynate, using approximately the same cooling and heating

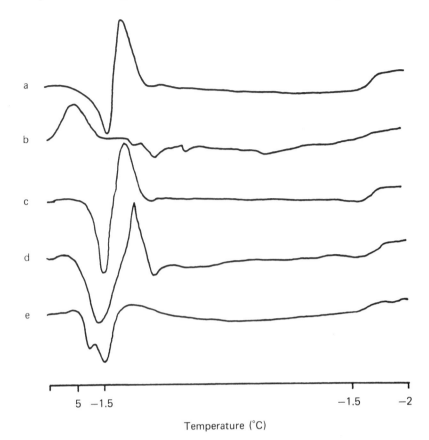

Fig. 1 — DTA profiles of 0.5% w/w aqueous solutions of sodium ethacrynate under selected cooling and heating conditions.

Sample	Cooled to (°C)	Cooling rate (°C min−1)	Heating rate (°C min−1)
a	−140	20	1.5
b	−50	0.5	0.2
c	−45	1.5	1.5
d	−140	1.5	1.5
e	−140	20	0.2

rates, but the plateau temperature, where the shallow endotherm occurred, was found to be −0.8°C compared with −1.5°C found for the solution containing 0.5% w/w sodium ethacrynate. A slow cooled sample of the solution containing 2% w/w sodium ethacrynate showed a similar profile to that of a solution containing 0.5% sodium ethacrynate with no apparent liquidus curve but a large exotherm between −0.7°C and 5°C on warming. For all the samples containing 2% w/w sodium ethacrynate, a gradual decrease in resistance was noted starting between −8°C and −12°C up to the point where the shallow DTA endotherm started, at which time a rapid decrease in resistance was observed.

Both the DTA and EC profiles of a solution containing 4% w/w sodium ethacrynate rapidly cooled to $-140°C$ and heated at $-1.5°C\,min^{-1}$ indicated a transition occurring between $-48°C$ and $-14°C$ as indicated by a shallow DTA endotherm and decrease in resistance (Fig. 2). An increase in resistance was then noted to $-8°C$ where it then began to decrease again.

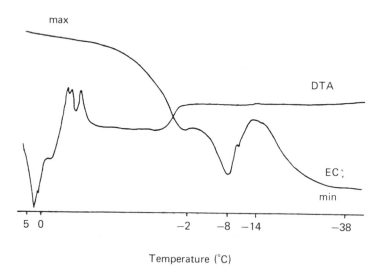

Fig. 2 — DTA and EC profiles of a 4% w/w aqueous solution of sodium ethacrynate cooled to $-140°C$ (20°C min-1) and warmed at 1.5°C.

Physical form and moisture content
X-ray powder diffraction patterns of the slow cooled and fast cooled freeze-dried sodium ethacrynate are shown in Fig. 3. Microscopical examination of the initial freeze-dried samples revealed relatively large plates of sodium ethacrynate present in those prepared from the more concentrated solutions and the large fill volumes. All the freeze-dried samples had a moisture content of less than 0.5% w/w.

Chemical stability
The loss of chemical integrity of sodium ethacrynate prepared by the fast-freezing process as a function of period of storage at 60°C is shown in Table 1. Stressed fast cooled samples partially or totally liquefied to produce a clear oil. Sodium ethacrynate freeze dried using the slow-freezing process retained greater than 95% if its initial potency after storage for 9 months at 60°C. The only significant degradation product observed using HPLC was identified as ethacrynic acid dimer.

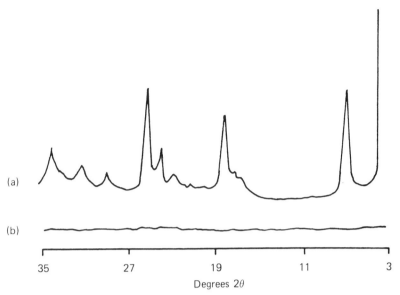

Fig. 3 — X-ray powder diffraction patterns of (a) slow cooled and (b) fast cooled
freeze-dried sodium ethacrynate.

DISCUSSION

The findings of the DTA and EC studies suggested that a variety of
amorphous and crystalline forms of sodium ethacrynate could be formed
dependent upon the concentrations of solute and the freezing conditions
employed during freeze drying. DTA profiles were generally similar and
showed a shallow endotherm followed by a sharp exotherm. Such a profile is
typical of a glass transition of a compound followed by its crystallization. A
glass transition may be defined as the passage from a vitreous state to a
highly viscous supercooled liquid. Crystallization is the passage from the
amorphous to the crystalline state. When the 'glass' is warmed it changes
into a supercooled liquid where the water molecules undergo rotational and
translational motion in addition to the vibrational motion found in the glassy
state. The temperature at which this transition occurs will depend on the
nature and concentration of the solute and the interaction between solute
and water molecules. As the temperature is increased further the molecules
acquire sufficient mobility to pass from the amorphous state to the ordered
structure of a crystal. The EC profiles of the solutions containing 0.5% w/w
sodium ethacrynate were in agreement with this hypothesis. A gradual
decrease in resistance corresponding to the time of the shallow endotherm
and increase or plateau in resistance noted at the time of the exotherm
supported the hypothesis of glass transition and crystallization. The solutions containing 2% w/w sodium ethacrynate and similar DTA profiles to
those containing 0.5% w/w sodium ethacrynate. The EC profiles of the
solutions were also similar but a very gradual decrease in resistance on

Table 1 — The percentage (±S.D.) of fast cooled freeze-dried sodium ethacrynate remaining after storage at 60°C for selected periods of time

Fill volume (ml)	Days	Concentration of sodium ethacrynate (%w/v) in initial solutions			
		1	2	3	4
0.5	15	95.3 (0.6)	97.7 (0.6)	98.3 (0.6)	98.7 (0.6)
	30	82.7 (0.6)	92.0 (1.0)	93.7 (0.6)	94.7 (0.6)
	45	65.3 (3.0)	78.3 (4.0)	85.3 (3.0)	90.0 (1.0)
	60	42.3 (5.0)	62.0 (2.0)	73.7 (4.2)	79.3 (2.1)
1.0	15	98.7 (0.6)	98.7 (0.6)	99.3 (0.6)	99.3 (0.6)
	30	93.7 (1.5)	94.2 (1.2)	95.3 (0.6)	96.3 (0.6)
	45	85.0 (2.6)	88.7 (1.5)	89.7 (1.5)	92.7 (1.2)
	60	72.0 (4.6)	82.3 (2.1)	84.3 (1.5)	87.7 (0.6)
2.0	15	98.7 (0.6)	98.3 (0.6)	98.7 (0.6)	99.0 (0.0)
	30	93.7 (0.6)	94.3 (1.2)	92.8 (2.0)	93.0 (1.0)
	45	87.0 (3.0)	90.7 (0.6)	85.0 (3.0)	85.7 (1.2)
	60	77.0 (4.0)	83.0 (1.0)	74.3 (2.5)	78.0 (2.0)
3.0	15	98.3 (0.6)	98.7 (0.6)	99.3 (0.6)	99.7 (0.6)
	30	94.3 (0.6)	92.3 (1.5)	94.0 (0.0)	96.0 (1.0)
	45	88.7 (1.5)	86.0 (2.0)	86.7 (1.5)	92.3 (0.6)
	60	78.7 (5.5)	74.7 (2.5)	76.7 (4.5)	84.0 (1.0)

warming from approximately −12°C was noted in the 2% w/w solutions, suggesting some melting or glass transition event occurring, however this was not apparent from the DTA trace. The DTA and EC profiles of a solution containing 4% w/w sodium ethacrynate was more complex and the transition between −38° and −14°C was considered to be another glass transition followed by crystallization between −14° and −8°C. A further glass transition and crystallization was indicated by the decrease in resistance noted between −8°C and −2°C. The thermal events occurring on heating above −2°C were as described for the solutions containing 0.5% and 2% w/w sodium ethacrynate. The presence of glass transitions in the frozen solutions indicated that dependent upon the freezing conditions employed during the freeze-drying cycle, crystalline or amorphous material may be obtained. The differences in X-ray diffraction patterns for the freeze-dried samples revealed that crystalline material was obtained by the slow-freezing process and amorphous material by the fast-freezing process.

Stability of freeze-dried sodium ethacrynate prepared in vials and sealed under vacuum was assessed for degradation after storage at 60°C for selected periods of time. This sealing procedure ensured that samples were studied under low humidity conditions preventing crystallization of amorphous material present within the samples. Stability of the 'slow frozen' crystalline material was superior to that found for any of the 'fast frozen' amorphous samples and indicated that the physical form influences the chemical stability of sodium ethacrynate.

On the basis of the known degradation mechanism of sodium ethacrynate in solution [3], second order degradation kinetics were anticipated. However a superficial examination of the loss of sodium ethacrynate with time indicated that degradation proceeded at an ever increasing rate over the time period studied. Sodium ethacrynate dimer was the only significant degradate observed suggesting that it was the apparent rate of reaction that was changing and not an additional degradation pathway operating. The observation that the dimer was produced as an oil in samples of amorphous freeze-dried sodium ethacrynate provided an explanation of the increasing apparent rate of reaction.

Stability is dependent upon both the concentration of the solute and the fill volume employed. For fill volumes of 0.5 and 1 ml, least degradation was noted in preparations freeze dried from solutions containing 4% w/w sodium ethacrynate. For these fill volumes, stability gradually decreased with decreasing concentration of the solutions used to prepare the samples. For the 2 ml and 3 ml fill volumes stability did not appear to be a function of concentration.

It would be expected from the known characteristics of the system that the larger fill volumes will take longer to freeze and visual observation of the freezing of samples during the freeze drying process confirmed this. For 0.5 ml fill volume, freezing was almost instantaneous, whereas for the 1, 2 and 3 ml fill volumes complete freezing took up to several minutes. This additional time in the solution phase and the greater temperature gradients present may allow some of the sodium ethacrynate to freeze in the crystalline form, or in the case of the more concentrated solutions, allow crystalline sodium ethacrynate to be precipitated as the equilibrium solubility is known to decrease with decreasing temperature. Precipitation of crystalline plates of sodium ethacrynate in many of the higher fill volume samples was confirmed by microscopy, however a quantitative assessment of the extent of precipitation could not be made, thus the final solution concentration immediately prior to freezing was not known. The complex interacting pattern of events occurring during freezing allowed an explanation of the inconsistent profiles of loss of ethacrynate acid with time observed in the higher fill volume (2 and 3 ml) samples.

REFERENCES

[1] W. B. Hagerman, F. A. Bacher, M. G. Coady, E. M. Cohen, P. R. Damn, R. Roman and J. A. Ryan, Annual Spring Meeting, A.Ph.A., Montreal, Canada (1978).

[2] A. J. Phillips, Ph.D. Thesis, C.N.A.A., Brighton (1978).

[3] R. J. Yarwood, A. J. Phillips, N. A. Dickinson and J. H. Collett, *Drug Dev. Ind. Pharm.*, **9** 35 (1983).
[4] R. J. Yarwood, W. D. Moore and J. H. Collett, *J. Pharm. Sci.*, **74**, 220 (1985).

4

The stability of drug adsorbates on to silica

Rolf Daniels, Bernhard Kerstiens, Helga Tischinger-Wagner
and **Herbert Rupprecht**
Department of Pharmaceutical Technology, Institute of Pharmacy,
University of Regensburg, Regensburg, West Germany

SUMMARY

Colloidal and porous silicas are used as carriers in solid, semi-solid and liquid dosage forms. Adsorption of active ingredients on to their large surface areas can be used to regulate drug release or for the uniform distribution of drug in single dose units with a very low drug content. The contact between drug and carrier surface on the molecular level can be of great importance for the chemical stability of drug preparations and this can be demonstrated by the following examples.

Hydrolytic degradation of acetyl salicylic acid in dry silica adsorbates is mainly determined by alkaline impurities of the carrier and amount of water adsorbed on to the silica surface. The 'catalytic' action of silicas is, therefore, directly dependent on the preparation technique of the carrier. Propantheline, a cationic ester compound, is adsorbed on to silica from aqueous solution. In aqueous silica suspensions and in dry adsorbates, the ester hydrolysis is controlled by the pH, the neutral salt content and buffer substances, due to different adsorption mechanisms.

The oxidative degradation of butylhydroxyanisole in silica adsorbates was also found to be enhanced in the presence of alkaline impurities. The oxidation of linoleic acid methylester in oleogels of colloidal silica proved to be influenced both by carrier impurities and the specific adsorption of intermediates (peroxides) on to the surface.

INTRODUCTION

The concept of drug deposition on insoluble hydrophilic inorganic carriers is of great interest both in terms of the controlled enhancement of drug dissolution rate and a uniform distribution of low dosed drugs in single-dose application forms [1,2]. Silica is of outstanding importance as a carrier material for this purpose, due to its excellent physicochemical and physiological properties and the large specific surfaces of colloidal and porous silica preparations available for drug deposition [3].

Single drug molecules are uniformly distributed over the surface of the silica and bound to specific adsorption sites. The stability of the drug may, however, be influenced by the catalytic action of the active surface sites of the carrier; impurities of the excipient or adsorbed water at the solid surface. At surface coverages of less than 100% each drug molecule is in contact with the carrier and simultaneously exposed to the atmosphere, allowing oxygen or water molecules to attack reactive sites directly from the gas phase.

The main aim of this work was to demonstrate specific features of some degradation processes on silica surfaces. Representative drug models were chosen which were sensitive to hydrolytic or oxidative actions. These were used to evaluate the influence of different particle and surface structures on the silica carriers.

MATERIALS

The silica carriers used were all of the hydrophilic amorphous type, characterized by reactive silanol groups on the surface and a non-reactive SiO_2 framework [4] (Table 1). The flame hydrolysed products Aerosil 200 (A 200) and HDK N 20 are composed of non-porous colloidal particles with traces of adsorbed HCl from the combustion of $SiCl_4$ [3]. Silicas produced by sol-gel transformation of Na-silicates — Syloid 244, KG 60 — are porous as well as being particulate and are obtained by hydrolytic polycondensation of polyethoxysiloxanes [5]. They contain impurities such as Na_2O, Fe_2O_3, Al_2O_3, or NH_3.

As examples of hydrolysable drugs, the esters acetylsalicylic acid (ASA) and propantheline bromide (Prop), a cationic aggregating drug, were selected. While ASA shows no adsorption from aqueous solution on to silica surfaces [6], Prop is strongly adsorbed from aqueous media [7]. Butyl-hydroxyanisole (BHA) was the drug model used to study the oxidative degradation of phenolic compounds in silica adsorbates. Autoxidation was monitored in silica suspensions of lineoleic acid methylester (LME) (Table 2).

PREPARATION OF THE ADSORBATES

Numerous references deal with the chemical stability of drugs, in which the drugs are deposited on the silica surface as crystals or thick amorphous layers [1,8,9]. The surface deposition technique used in these experiments,

Table 1 — Silica excipients

Product	Particle size	Pore size (nm)	Spec. surface ($m^2 g^{-1}$)	Method of manufacture	Impurities [%]				
					Na_2O	Fe_2O_3	Al_2O_3	HCl	NH_3
Aerosil 200[a] [A 200]	10–40 nm	Non-porous	220	Flame hydrolysis of $SiCl_4$	—	—	—	<0.004	—
HDK N 20[b]	5–30 nm	Non-porous	207	Flame hydrolysis of $SiCl_4$	—	—	—	<0.004	—
TK 900[a]	2–15 μm	Non-porous	160	Electric arc	0.007	0.093	0.100	/	—
Syloid 244[c]	~2 μm	18	480	Sol-Gel	0.136	0.012	0.185	/	—
Kr 36[d]	~1 mm	14	510	Hydrolytic polycondensation of polyethoxysiloxane	0.002	0.004	—	/	0.132
KG 60[e]	~0.5 mm	6	550	Sol-Gel	0.100	0.016	0.093	/	—

[a]DEGUSSA, Frankfurt a.M., West Germany, [b]Wacker Chemie, München, West Germany, [c]Grace, Worms, West Germany. [d]own development (e), [e]E. Merck, Darmstadt, West Germany.

Table 2 — Drug models

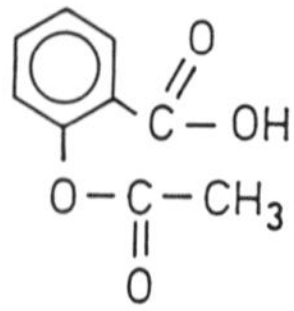

Acetylsalicylic acid
ASA

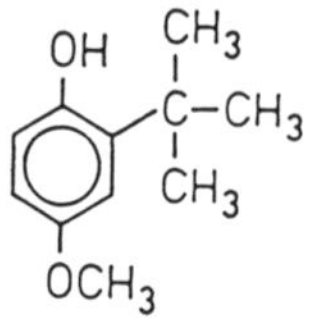

Butylhydroxyanisole
BHA

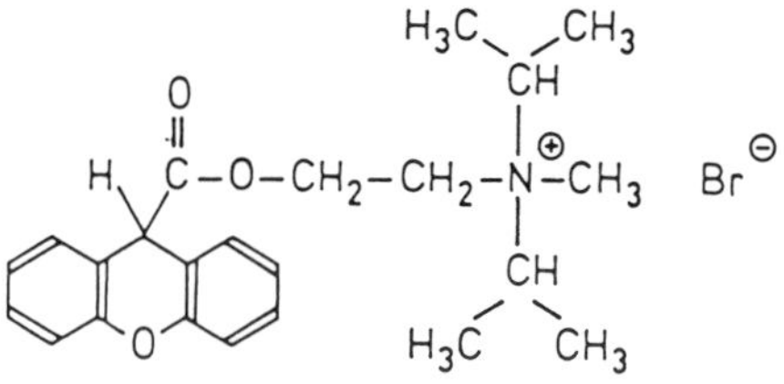

Propantheline bromide
Prop

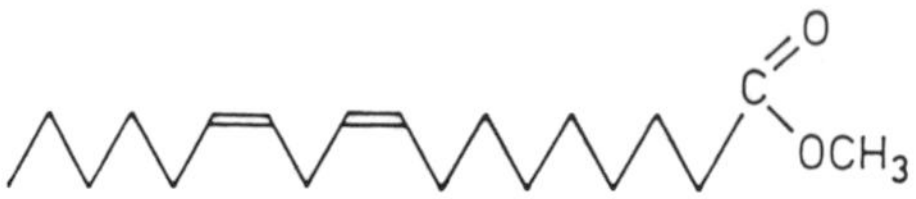

Linoleic acid methylester
LME

was different. Adsorption equilibria were established at the silica/solution interface by means of an appropriate solvent. By this technique well defined drug adsorbates on the silica carriers were obtained. In these adsorbates the position of the drug molecules on the carrier surface can be evaluated from adsorption data — surface coverage, heat of adsorption — and by IR and UV spectroscopy of the adsorbed molecules [4].

Acetylsalicylic acid (ASA)
ASA was adsorbed from dichlormethane solution on to the silicas by a standard procedure. After equilibration of the silica with the drug solution at 20°C (within 12 h), the adsorbates were removed from the liquid phase by

filtering or centrifugation and then dried in a vacuum. The dry adsorbates were stored over P_2O_5 and the initial contents of ASA and salicylic acid determined before starting the stability experiments.

In Fig. 1 the position of an ASA molecule in adsorbates on silica surfaces

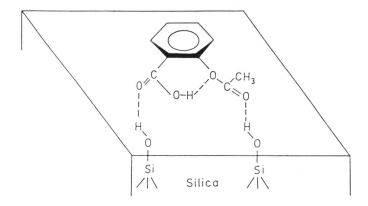

Fig. 1 — Structure of an acetyl salicylic acid molecule, adsorbed on the silica surface.

is given schematically. The drug is adsorbed by hydrogen bonds between surface silanol groups and proton acceptor groups of ASA, between the ester linkage or the π electron system of the ring. The adsorbate's structure was deduced from heats of adsorption — 17 kJ mol^{-1}, and IR spectra of the adsorbates [6]. In addition, strongly adsorbed water molecules are present in the drug adsorbates on the silica carriers.

Butylhydroxyanisole (BHA)

For the adsorption of BHA on to the silicas the same procedure was used, except that cyclohexane as solvent was employed. For the structure of the adsorbates it is supposed that the BHA molecules are flatly attached to the surface, fixed in this position by hydrogen bonds between the phenolic groups and the silanol groups of the silica (Fig. 2) [10].

Propantheline bromide (Prop)

In contrast to ASA and BHA, the aggregating cationic Prop was adsorbed from aqueous solution on to the silica surface (Fig. 3) [11]. Depending on the equilibrium concentration the Prop cations are primarily bound to the silica surface by ion exchange in the low concentration range (Fig. 3A) according to

$$\text{Prop}^+ + \equiv\text{Si–OH} \rightleftharpoons \equiv\text{Si–O Prop} + \text{H}^+$$

This mechanism is indicated by a decrease of pH in the supernatant aqueous phase during the establishment of the adsorption equilibrium (i.e. pH 4.5→ pH 3.8) and by the difference in counter-ion — Br$^-$ — binding.

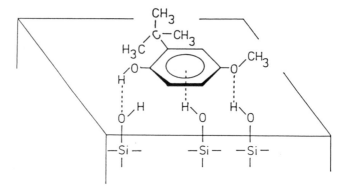

Fig. 2 — Structure of a 3-BHA-molecule, adsorbed on the silica surface.

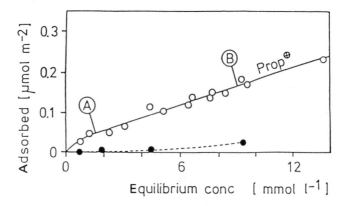

Adsorption isotherm

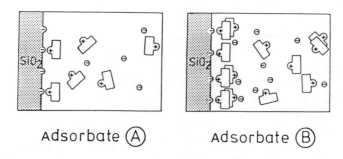

Adsorbate Ⓐ   Adsorbate Ⓑ

Fig. 3 — Structures of propantheline adsorbates on the silica surface, depending on
the adsorption equilibrium.

At higher concentrations Prop cations are adsorbed by hydrophobic bonding to the primary bound species which are themselves orientated perpendicular to the surface (Fig. 3B). These Prop cations are accompanied to a great extent by their counter-ions, Br^-, according to the concept of hemimicelle binding of surfactants [12].

The adsorption of Prop at the silica surface can be improved by increasing the pH and thereby increasing the cation exchange or by the addition of neutral salts with water structure-breaking counter-ions of Prop, such as nitrate [7]. This effect can be attributed to an enhancement of ion pair adsorption, as controlled by hydrophobic and electrostatic interactions. Consequently the Prop ions are orientated with their polar head groups to the silica surface in the ion exchange layer. The secondarily attached Prop are orientated with their quaternary ammonium groups to the aqueous phase, with some of the counter-ions in close contact (in the Stern-layer) and some of them in the diffuse part of the electical double layer at the interface.

HYDROLYSIS OF ESTER COMPOUNDS

Acetylsalicylic acid adsorbates

The loss of ASA in adsorbates on different silica carriers stored under 'open storage conditions' [13] at 21°C and 31% relative humidity (RH) is shown in Fig. 4. It can be seen that a significant order of rank occurs. The lowest rate of hydrolysis is observed on HDK N 20, followed by A 200 with a moderate stability for ASA, both being flame-hydrolysed non-porous colloidal silicas. In contrast, the colloidal non-porous TK 900 as well as the porous KG 60 H show the strongest catalytic action on ASA degradation. The porous silicas Kr 36 and Syloid 244 are characterized by intermediate degradation rates of ASA.

This order of catalytic action of the silica carriers on ASA hydrolysis is obviously more dependant on the sum of the catalytic impurities on their surfaces (i.e. Na_2O, Al_2O_3, NH_3) than on their structural characteristics (particle size, porosity, silanol group density). According to Edwards [14] the ASA degradation rate constant k is related to the OH^- concentration in an aqueous environment by

$$k = k' [OH^-]$$

In the silica-ASA adsorbates an adsorption equilibrium also exists between water in the gas phase and on the silica surface. The adsorbed H_2O can react with alkaline impurities deposited on the silica surface present as $NaHCO_3$ and/or Na_2CO_3. Hydrolysis of these compounds releases OH-ions which then attack the ester linkages of adsorbed ASA molecules. Adsorbed NH_3 serves in the same way as an OH^- ion source.

In contrast, surface bound HCl and Al_2O_3 (the latter being a Brönsted centre when adsorbed on SiO_2) can produce H_3O^+ ions with the adsorbed water, thus stimulating an acidic catalysed ester hydrolysis [15].

These conclusions are supported by the direct correlation between the ASA hydrolysis-rates and the relative humidities of the storage conditions

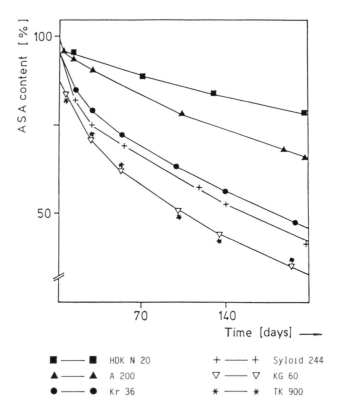

Fig. 4 — Hydrolysis of ASA in adsorbates on different silicas (21°C±0.5; 32% RH; θ=1).

which determine the water 'supply' in the adsorbates. From Fig. 5 it is clearly seen that ASA degradation is continuously accelerated by increasing the relative humidity when using the non-porous HDK N 20 as a support. For the porous Kr 36 silica the rate of ASA-degradation shows a maximum value at 86% RH (Fig. 6). This can be explained by capillary condensation at higher RH values (i.e. 98%), thereby filling the silica pores with aqueous media. In the presence of a liquid water phase a quite different situation exists. Dissolution of silica, dilution effects as well as the influence of water structure phenomena must now be considered as influencing ASA decomposition [16].

The mechanism of ASA hydrolysis in adsorbates on silica surfaces can now be discussed in detail, considering the amount of water molecules on the surface which are available for ester hydrolysis. At 0% RH the porous Kr 36 adsorbate contains 7.3% H_2O, which corresponds to one H_2O molecule on each surface silanol group. Therefore the ratio between adsorbed ASA and water molecules is 1:10. To establish a closely packed water monolayer on the silica surface, RH values >60% are necessary. Even

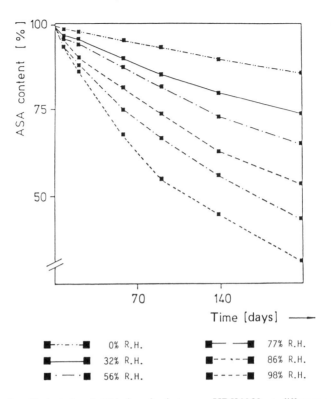

Fig. 5 — Hydrolysis of ASA in adsorbates on HDK N 20 at different relative humidities (21°C±0.5; θ=1).

in a water vapour saturated atmosphere, the amount of adsorbed water on the ASA adsorbates is far distant from forming 'solution layers'. On HDK N 20 the ratio is 1:400 and on Kr 36, 1:150. For comparison, the ratio between ASA and water molecules in a saturated aqueous solution is 1:2500 at 21°C [17].

It is therefore concluded that the diffusion rate of water molecules on the silica surface and/or OH^- and H_3O^+ ions, are the rate determining factors for ASA hydrolysis. It is here assumed that at room temperature only water molecules are able to migrate on the surface, while ASA molecules essentially remain on their adsorption sites. This view of ASA hydrolysis is confirmed by the strong correlation observed between the rate constant of ASA degradation and the water content of the adsorbates, based on second order kinetics [17].

Propantheline-adsorbates
Considering the stability of propantheline (Prop) on silica surfaces, there is a different stress on the drug during the production of the adsorbates, compared with ASA. In contrast to the adsorption of ASA from dichlor-

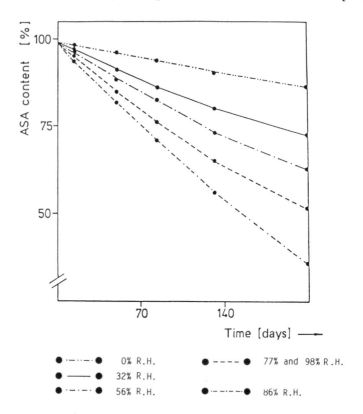

Fig. 6 — Hydrolysis of ASA in adsorbates on Kr 36 at different humidities
(21°C±0.5; θ=1).

methane solution where water can be sufficiently excluded, the adsorbates of Prop are formed from aqueous solutions. Therefore hydrolytic degradation and adsorption become parallel processes in these systems.

In Fig. 7, Prop decomposed to a quaternary ammonium alcohol and xanthene carboxylic acid is shown during the preparation phase of adsorbates on Kr 36 by dotted lines. Taking the adsorbates obtained from aqueous solutions of Prop as a standard (pH ~ 6), the influence of different additives, which may serve to enhance the adsorption, is clearly seen. In the presence of a phosphate buffer (pH 6) the degradation rate remains the same as in pure aqueous solutions. Change of the pH to 7.6 by addition of NaOH, accelerates the propantheline decomposition due to an increased concentration of catalytic OH ions. An unexpected low degradation rate is observed in the presence of $NaNO_3$. Different effects may contribute to the better stability of Prop in the presence of this inorganic electrolyte. NO_3^- ions, counter-ions of $Prop^+$ as well as Br^- and OH^-, may displace the catalytic active hydroxyl ions from the diffuse electrical double layer at the adsorbate–solution interface and, particularly, in the Stern layer of the

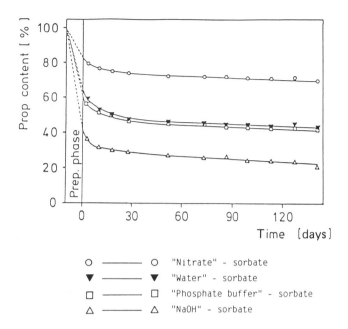

Fig. 7 — Hydrolysis of propantheline in adsorbates on Kr 36, prepared in the presence of different additives (21°C ± 0.5; 0% RH).

adsorbate. It should also be considered that the amount of Prop adsorbed by hydrophobic interactions to the primarily bound Prop cations is increased by the NO_3^- ions. These Prop ions are orientated to the aqueous phase and may be prevented from coming into close contact with the silica surface [7]. This portion of the adsorbed Prop is, therefore, not available as a substrate for the catalytic action of silica surface groups.

After removing the adsorbates from the aqueous dispersion and drying them (*in vacuo*), they were stored over P_2O_5, corresponding to 0% RH at 21°C. A residue of 7% strongly adsorbed H_2O remains under these conditions in Kr 36-Prop adsorbates. Within the first three weeks of storage the hydrolysis of Prop in each of the adsorbates is chracterized by an initial phase with high degradation rates, followed then by a period of an almost constant, considerably lower rate (full lines in Fig. 7).

At the beginning of the storage period the ratio 1:11 between adsorbed drug and water molecules on the silica surface is of the same order as that with ASA adsorbates. At 0% RH there exists no supply of water for the hydrolysis of the drug from the gas phase. Water, which is used by the hydrolysis process, must come to the sites of action — the ester group. This water transport becomes again the rate determining factor for the hydrolysis reaction, while the additives, very important in aqueous dispersions, are of minor importance.

The degradation of Prop is accelerated if the adsorbates on silica are exposed to a storage climate with an increased relative himidity (Fig. 8). Adsorbates prepared from pure aqueous solutions and from phosphate buffer are characterized by the same order of decomposition rate at 35% RH (dotted range Fig. 8 and RH >76%, hatched range Fig. 8). As expected in 'NaOH' adsorbates higher degradation rates are observed (dotted lines), but the differences are smaller than in aqueous silica suspensions [7] and not so pronounced as in adsorbates of ASA on silica with the same content of NaOH. Adsorbates, prepared in the presence of $NaNO_3$ show the most substantial enhancement of the Prop hydrolysis rate if the RH is increased (Fig. 8 hatched–dotted lines).

Summarizing, the hydrolysis of Prop in silica adsorbates is characterized by the following features. The decomposition rates are strongly dependent upon the relative humidities of storage and, consequently, on the water content of the adsorbates. Transport of water to and on the surface is proposed to be the rate determining process.

From the specific degradation rates of the adsorbates found in the presence of different additives it seems apparent that Prop in direct contact with the silica surface decomposes faster than Prop adsorbed in the hemi-micellar state, and therefore orientated with the polar groups to the aqueous phase. Compared to ASA adsorbates contaminated with alkaline impurities, the Prop adsorbates are not so sensitive to hydrolytic action upon the addition of NaOH.

From these results it is concluded that Prop cations are catalysed in their hydrolysis by adsorptive interaction with the silica surface. Bound by the electrostatic forces between the quaternary ammonium groups and negatively charged adsorption sites on the silica surface they establish additional hydrogen bonds between the ester carbonyl groups and surface silanols (Fig. 9). This can be concluded from IR measurements of the adsorbates [17].

As a consequence, the carbonium state of the ester linkage may be stabilized by these adsorptive interactions. In this way the attack of hydroxyl ions — the rate determining step of ester hydrolysis in aqueous solution (S_{N2}-reaction) — is facilitated [15]. An increased number of dissociated silanol groups at higher pH-values (after addition of NaOH) increases the number of ion exchange sites, but diminishes the number of silanol groups acting as proton donors for hydrogen bonding. This explains the relative insensitivity of the Prop adsorbates to alkali in comparison to ASA adsorbates. Adsorption in the presence of $NaNO_3$ means that most of the adsorbed Prop species are not in the correct position to allow these two adsorption mechanisms and therefore they show better stability.

OXIDATIVE DEGRADATION

Butylhydroxyanisole (BHA)

The antioxidant BHA was chosen as a sensitive model for studying oxidative degradation in silica adsorbates. After reaction with oxygen, dibenzofuran

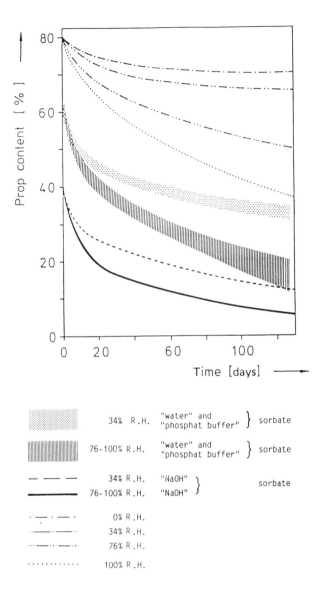

Fig. 8 — Propantheline hydrolysis in adsorbates on silica Kr 36. Influence of preparation (21°C±0.5).

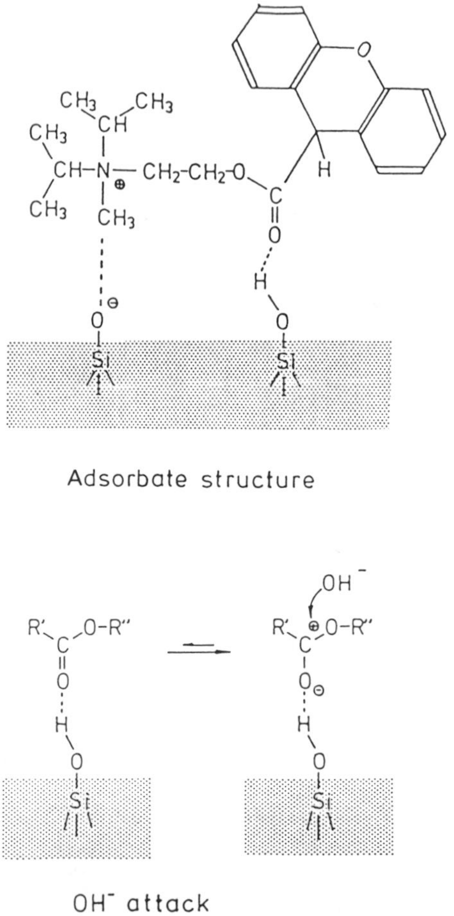

Adsorbate structure

OH⁻ attack

Fig. 9 — Propantheline adsorbate on the silica surface: Interaction by electrostatic forces and hydrogen bonding; attack of the OH⁻ ion at the ester group.

chinone is finally formed, with phenoxiradicals and a diphenol as intermediates (Fig. 10) [18,19]. The loss of BHA was monitored by amperometric determination of the BHA content of the adsorbates [20].

In Fig. 11 the degradation of BHA in adsorbates on different silicas stored at 21°C and 37% RH are shown. With the exception of Syloid 244 the silicas do not significantly influence the oxidation of adsorbed BHA. Any catalytic effect of the silica surface can therefore be excluded. The different BHA stability in Syloid 244 adsorbates is attributed to the high content of impurities (Table 1) on the carrier, which act as catalysts in the oxidation process [21].

By increasing the RH an opposite effect is observed on 'clean', low contaminated silicas and on Syloid 244. In adsorbates on colloidal A 200 and

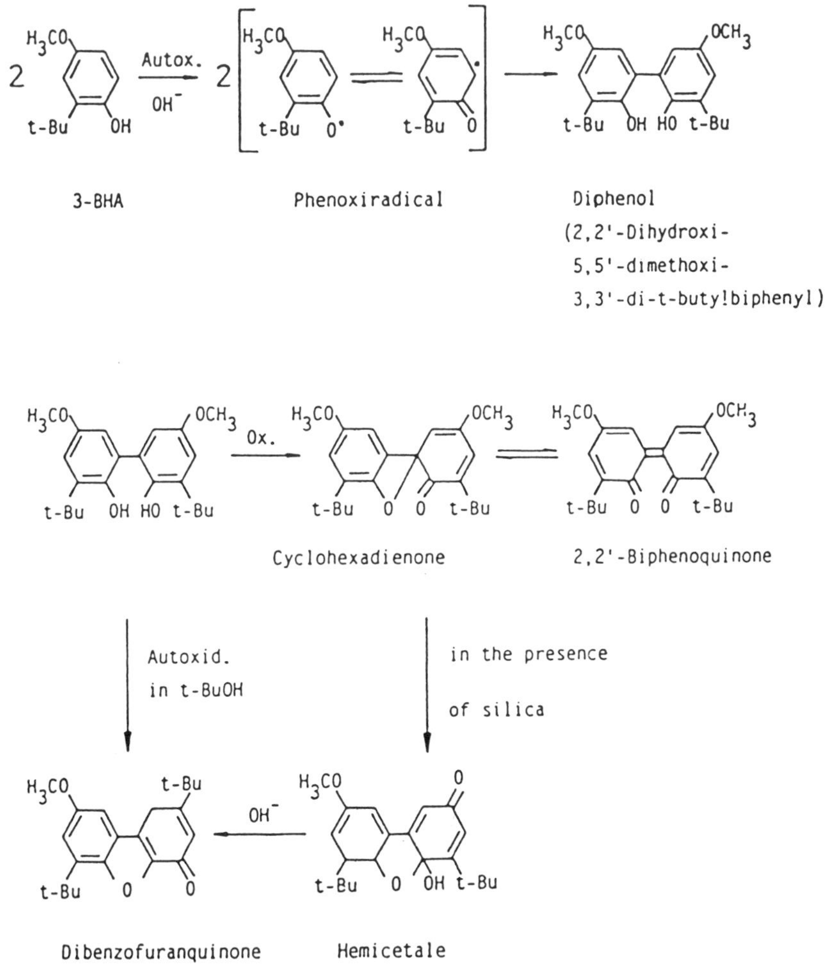

Fig. 10 — Course of 3-BHA degradation.

porous Kr 36 (both silicas with a low content of impurities), the oxidation is accelerated if RH values are established >76% (Fig. 12). This can be explained by a progressive adsorption of the transport medium water on the surface.

On the Syloid 244 surface, however, increasing amounts of adsorbed water (corresponding RH >80%) are accompanied by decreasing reaction rates for BHA oxidation (Fig. 13). The most outstanding difference in impurity content is the relatively high content of Al_2O_3. It is supposed that in the presence of higher amounts of water, the surface-bound alumina may progressively act as Brönsted centres, generating H_3O^+ ions which reduce the surface pH in the adsorbates. Consequently, the stability of BHA is improved [20].

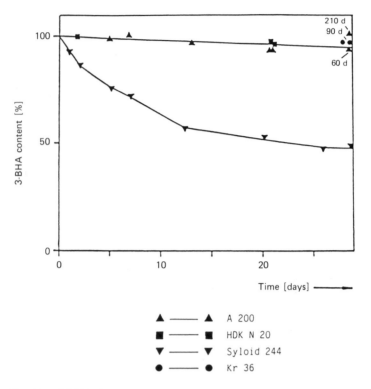

Fig. 11 — 3-BHA degradation in adsorbates in different silica-carriers (20°C ± 0.5; 32% RH).

Linoleic acid methylester (LME)

In addition to the stability studies of different drug molecules on silica surfaces in dry adsorbates, the action of silica in contact with liquid LME should be outlined in brief. Following the autoxidation of LME in suspensions of different silicas (6%), by measuring the oxygen consumption characteristic differences are obtained (Fig. 14). The silicas are obviously promoting the autoxidation of the unsaturated compound, with the non-porous colloidal A 200 being the most effective catalyst, followed by Syloid 244 (with a high content of Fe_2O_3). Kr 36 exhibits the lowest catalytic action.

The enhancement of LME oxidation in the presence of silica is explained by adsorption of the reaction intermediates — the peroxides — on to the surface, which are then activated in the adsorbed state [20]. Also taking into consideration the significant influence of metal impurities as catalysts, the different action of porous and non-porous silicas is obviously due to the slow transport processes inside the porous particles.

Summarizing, hydrolytic degradation is stimulated by basic as well as by acidic impurities, with the alkaline impurities being the most effective by

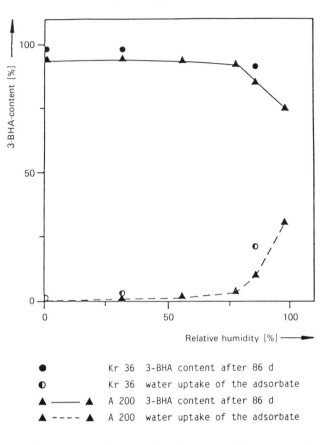

Fig. 12 — 3-BHA degradation in SiO$_2$ adsorbates at different relative humidities
(20°C ± 0.5; θ = 0.5).

generating OH ions with adsorbed water. The hydrolytic action of impurities is enhanced by increasing amounts of adsorbed water, which in turn is dependent on the atmospheric relative humidity.

Strong adsorption from aqueous media — i.e. by electrostatic interactions — provokes catalytic action of the silica surface on the hydrolysis of ester compounds by direct interactions between silanol groups and the ester groups. Molecules missing these strong electrostatic actions are desorbed in aqueous dispersion from the silica and therefore a catalytic action is restricted to impurities, generating OH$^-$ or H$_3$O$^+$.

Oxidative processes such as phenol oxidation can also be stimulated by impurities, especially by a combination of alkaline and heavy metal oxides. Autoxidation of unsaturated compounds is catalysed by an adsorption of the reaction intermediates — the peroxides — on to the silica surface.

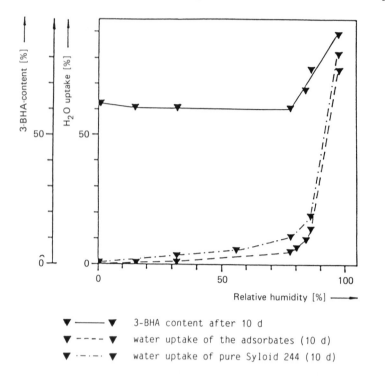

Fig. 13 — 3-BHA degradation in Syloid 244 adsorbates at different relative humidities ($20°C \pm 0.5$; $\theta = 0.5$).

ACKNOWLEDGEMENTS

Propantheline Bromide was kindly supplied by Searle Pharmaceuticals, Northumberland, UK, and the porous silica by Professor Dr K. Unger, University of Mainz, West Germany. This study was supported by the Fond der Chemischen Industrie and the Deutsche Forschungsgemeinschaft.

REFERENCES

[1] N. K. Jain and R. P. Kothari, *Indian Drugs,* **22**, 1 (1984).
[2] H. Rupprecht, *Acta Pharm. Technol.,* **26**, 13 (1980).
[3] H. Rupprecht and B. Kerstiens, *Pharm. Ztg,* **126**, 336 (1981).
[4] R. K. Iler, *The Chemisty of Silica.* J. Wiley & Sons, New York, Chichester, Brisbane, Toronto (1979).
[5] K. K. Unger and B. Scharf, *J. Colloid Interf. Sci.,* **55**, 377 (1976).
[6] H. Rupprecht and B. Kerstiens, *Pharm. Ztg,* **126**, 832 (1981).
[7] R. Daniels and H. Rupprecht, *Pharm. Res.,* **4**, 170 (1985).

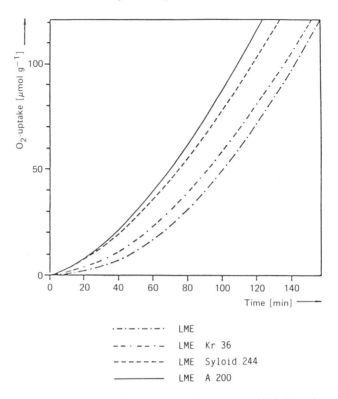

Fig. 14 — Oxygen uptake of linoleic acid methylester-SiO_2 (6%) dispersions during autoxidation, when exposed to UV-light (25°C ± 0.005; p_{O_2} = 213 mbar).

[8] D. C. Monkhouse and L. van Campen, *Drug Develop. Ind. Pharm.*, **10**, 1175 (1984).

[9] W. Loewe, M. Soliva and P. Speiser, *Pharm. Ind.*, **43**, 178 (1981).

[10] H. Tischinger-Wagner and H. Rupprecht, *Pharm. Ind.*, **46**, 275 (1984).

[11] H. Ferch, *Pharm. Ind.*, **41**, 186 (1979).

[12] D. W. Fuerstenau, *Pure Applied Chem.*, **24**, 135 (1970).

[13] H. Rupprecht and B. Kerstiens, *Pharm. Ztg*, **131**, in press (1986).

[14] L. J. Edwards, *Trans. Faraday Soc.*, **46**, 723 (1950); ibid., **47**, 1191 (1951); ibid., **48**, 696 (1952).

[15] J. Hine, *Reaktivität und Mechanismus in der organischen Chemie*, G. Thieme, Stuttgart, 1966.

[16] K. Klier and A. C. Zettlemoyer, *J. Colloid Interf. Sci.*, **58**, 216 (1977).

[17] B. Kerstiens and H. Rupprecht, *Pharm. Ztg*, **131**, in press (1986).

[18] F. R. Hegwill and S. L. Lee, *J. Chem. Soc. C*, 1549 (1968).

[19] H. Mauser and B. Nickel, *Angew. Chem.*, **77**, 378 (1965).

[20] L. Foley and F. M. Kimmerle, *Anal. Chem.*, **51**, 818 (1979).

[21] K. Thoma, *Arzneimittelstabilität*, Frankfurt a.M. 1980.

5

A preliminary investigation of a novel series of silica gels

G. N. Shah and **M. J. Groves,**
Department of Pharmaceutics, College of Pharmacy, University of Illinois at Chicago, 833 South Wood Street, Chicago, Illinois 60612, USA

SUMMARY

Silica gels may be produced by the hydrolytic polycondensation of organic silicates such as tetraethyl ortho silicate (TEOS) under appropriate conditions. These systems are of interest to the ceramic industry for making high purity silicate glasses at low temperatures. These silica gels may have application as drug delivery systems.

The gelation rates due to the hydrolytic polycondensation process depend on the concentration of TEOS and water, the temperature, and the presence of acid or base catalysts. A wide variety of polymeric silica gels having different polymeric matrices and pore sizes are possible. Of the alcohols and glycols screened for silica gel formulation, ethanol and glycerol appear to have a unique role in the gelation process although they do not appear to contribute directly to the hydrolytic polycondensation process.

INTRODUCTION

Silica gels may be produced by hydrolytic polycondensation of organic silicates under appropriate conditions. These systems are of significant interest to the ceramic industry since high purity silicate glasses may be made at low temperatures by a sol-gel process [1,2]. Drugs may be incorporated in these silica gels and other investigators have demonstrated the potential application of desicated silica gels as drug delivery systems [3]. Several drugs have been shown to act as a catalyst in the silica gel formation from an organic silicate, tetraethyl ortho silicate (TEOS) [3].

The preparation of silica gels from TEOS is currently being investigated at the University of Illinois as inexpensive transdermal vehicles or as oral drug delivery systems. TEOS undergoes hydrolytic polycondensation in the presence of water and ethanol as a mutual solvent under acidic or basic conditions. The sol-gel process can be categorized into three stages as follows:

(1) hydrolysis of alkoxide to form silanols
(2) condensation of the silanols to form siloxane bonds
(3) linking of the polymers to form rigid silica gels.

The relative process rates of the above stages are very much dependent on whether acid or base catalysts are used, the concentration of water and TEOS, and the temperature. Although all the silica gels formed from TEOS undergo the above three stages, the relative reaction rates and reaction mechanism for acid or base catalysed gels appear to be entirely different. Hydrolysis and condensation of TEOS in general may be summarized as follows:

$$\equiv SiOEt + H_2O \xrightarrow{\ OH^- \ or \ H^+\ } \equiv SiOH + EtOH$$

$$2 \equiv SiOH \xrightarrow{\hspace{2cm}} \equiv SiOSi \equiv + H_2O$$

A separate reaction mechanism was proposed for acid and base catalysed reactions by Keefer [4] and by Klein and Garvey [5]. Their proposed mechanisms were also supported by the H' NMR study of these systems by Assink and Kay [6].

EXPERIMENTAL

Materials

Tetraethyl orthosilicate (TEOS), gold label, Aldrich Chemical Company, Milwaukee, Wisconsin, USA. TEOS is a colourless hygroscopic liquid with a mild ester-like odour, boiling point of 168°C, freezing point of -77°C and flash point of 125°F. Prior to use, TEOS was distilled at 168°C and stored under nitrogen. *Glycerol*, gold label, Aldrich Chemical Co. *Hydrochloric acid and ammonium hydroxide*, Fisher Scientific Co. Ethyl alcohol (95%) and all other chemicals were obtained either from Aldrich or from Fisher.

Methods
Three types of phase diagrams were prepared.

(a) With water, TEOS and ethanol (95%)
(b) With glycerol replacing portions of water, TEOS and ethanol (95%) and
(c) Using other alcohols such as methyl and isopropyl (in place of ethyl), water and TEOS.

Sample preparation

Sample preparation involved a single step process in contrast to a two-step process used by other investigators [3,7,8]. Twenty points were selected (Fig. 1) on the miscible region of the phase diagram after initial screening of

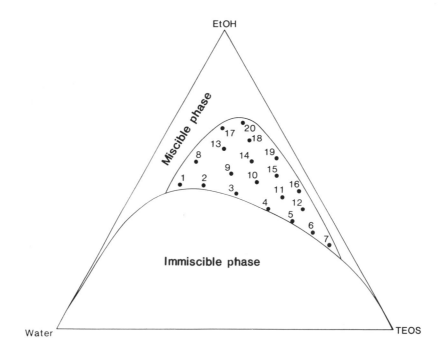

Fig. 1 — Phase diagram for TEOS, water and ethanol system.

gel formation in both the miscible and immiscible regions. Compositions were by weight in screw-capped glass vials. Acid or base catalysts in concentrations of 10^{-2} M to 10^{-4} M were added at the end. Vials were placed in a Fisher Versa bath at 45°C or 70°C and observed for gelation.

Results and discussion

TEOS and water are almost completely imiscible with each other. An alcohol as a mutual solvent is required. Phase boundaries using water, TEOS and either methyl, ethyl or isopropyl alcohol were basically very similar and did not change significantly by the addition of glycerol or other polyhydric glycols (Fig. 1).

   In the initial studies, the gel formation was observed in the entire region of the phase diagram using both acid and base catalysts. In the immiscible region of the phase diagram, either the gels did not form for a long period of time (200 h), or, if they did, the resulting gels were not uniform. At lower concentrations of either TEOS or water, gelation time in excess of 200 h was encountered and was not evaluated.

Even though both acid and base catalysis involve hydrolytic polycondensation in general, the resulting gels were quite distinct in appearance. Base catalysed gels produced branched clusters and generally the polymer did not gel as a unit; large particles sedimenting from solution. Base catalysed gels were also opaque in nature, but were more brittle compared with acid catalysed gels. Acid catalysed reactions produce linear polymers and the polymers gel as a complete entity. The resulting gels were less brittle compared with base catalysed gels and were transparent and elegant in appearance. These differences can be attributed to the reaction mechanisms proposed by Keefer [4] and by Klein and Garvey [5] for acid and base catalysis. According to Keefer [4], alkaline hydrolysis involves nucleophilic attack of the hydroxide ion on silicon, whereas acid hydrolysis involves an electrophilic reaction mechanism.

For all of the above reasons. The investigations were restricted to acid catalysed systems in the miscible region of the phase diagram (Fig. 1). Visual gelation times for systems in the miscible region were observed at 45°C and 70°C. Three different concentrations of hydrochloric acid as catalyst were selected for water, ethanol and TEOS systems together with similar systems containing glycerol.

Different gelation times and patterns were noted for systems with and without glycerol (Figs. 2(a) and 2(b)). The boundaries shown for different

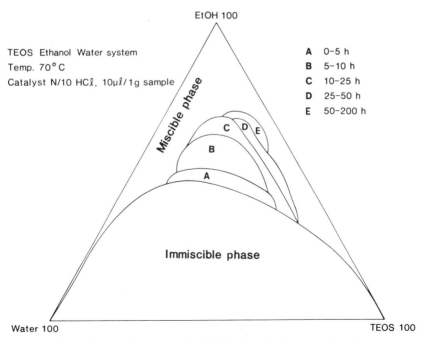

Fig. 2(a) — Gelation time pattern for TEOS, ethanol and water systems in presence of acid catalyst (HCl).

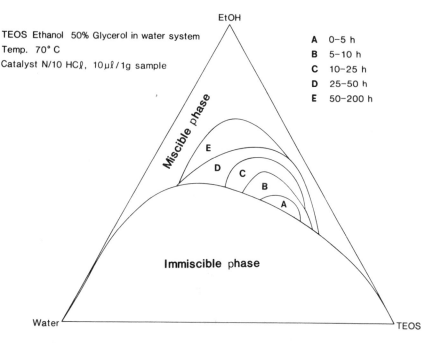

TEOS Ethanol 50% Glycerol in water system

Temp. 70° C

Catalyst N/10 HCℓ, 10μℓ/1g sample

A   0–5 h
B   5–10 h
C   10–25 h
D   25–50 h
E   50–200 h

EtOH

Miscible phase

Immiscible phase

Water   TEOS

Fig. 2(b) — Gelation time pattern for TEOS, ethanol and water systems containing glycerol in presence of acid catalyst (HCl).

regions A, B, C, D and E on the phase diagram (Figs 2(a) and 2(b)) were selected as approximate gelation times.

The presence of glycerol has a significant effect on the gelation time (Table 1). Gels were observed to form faster at low water/TEOS molar ratios in the presence of glycerol. In the absence of glycerol, gels formed faster at higher water/TEOS molar ratios (Table 1, Figs. 2(a) and 2(b)).

Gelation times for several polethylene and polypropylene glycols were also observed (Table 2). Gelation times with glycerol were less at those due to polyethylene and polypropylene glycols. Some of the gels formed with these glycols were also opaque. Some gels cracked and did not have the mechanical strength associated with the glycerol gels. Gelation times were found to be less than the higher temperature as might be anticipated (Table 3). Of the three acid catalyst (HCl) concentrations studied, gels formed faster at lower concentrations (Table 4).

Replacing ethyl alcohol with other alcohols had a significant effect on gelation process (Table 5). The gelation times were longer with the other alcohols and almost all the gels formed were opaque and did not possess the transparency observed with gels made with ethyl alcohol.

It is evident that gelation times have an impact on the nature and properties of the resulting gels. Not only does the concentration of water and TEOS affect the gelation process, but so also do the catalyst and tempera-

Table 1 — Gelation times in the presence and absence of glycerol

Location*	System A		System B		System C	
	Water/ TEOS molar ratio	GT	Water/ TEOS molar ratio	GT	Water/ TEOS molar ratio	GT
1	34.72	5:00	26.04	5:30	17.36	24:00
2	18.52	3:00	13.88	6:30	10.45	11:30
3	8.96	3:15	6.72	4:30	4.48	4:45
4	4.57	4:15	3.43	3:45	2.28	1:00
5	2.67	22:30	2.00	3:30	1.34	1:15
6	1.54	NG	1.15	45:00	0.77	NG
7	1.14	NG	0.65	NG	0.43	NG

* Location on phase diagram in Fig. 1.
System A — TEOS, ETOH and water system.
System B — TEOS, ETOH and (25% glycerol in water) system.
System C — TEOS, ETOH and (50% glycerol in water) system.
GT, gelation time in hours and minutes.
NG, no gel formation observed up to 200 h.
Conditions: Temperature 70°C. Catalyst, 0.1 N HCl, 10 μl/1.0 g sample.

Table 2 — Effect of other polyhydric glycols in place of glycerol

Type of polyhydric glycol	Gelation time (hours:min)
Glycerol	1:00
E-200	45:00
E-400	40:00
E-600	31:00
E-1000	27:00
E-4500	22:00
P-1200	19:00
P-2000	NG
P-4000	42:00

Sample: TEOS 43%, ETOH 40%, water 8.5%, glycol 8.5%.
E: Polyethylene glycol.
P: Polypropylene glycol.
NG: No gel formation observed up to 200 h.
Conditions: Temperature 70°C. Catalyst, 0.1 N HCl, 10 μl/1.0 g sample.

Table 3 — Effect of temperature on gelation time

Temp.	Gelation time (hours:min)				
	1*	2*	3*	4*	5*
45°C	37:00	6:30	11:20	20:30	50:00
70°C	5:00	3:30	3:15	4:15	22:30

* Location on phase diagram in Fig. 1.
Conditions: Catalyst 0.1 N HCl, 10 μl/1.0 g sample.

Table 4 — Gel formation at different acid catalyst (HCl) concentrations

*	Gelation time (hours:min)				
	1	2	3	4	5
Catalyst I	5:00	3:30	3:15	4:15	22:30
Catalyst II	28:00	21:30	10:30	18:00	44:00
Catalyst III	53:00	36:00	21:30	20:30	29:00

* Location of sample on phase diagram in Fig. 1.
I   contains 0.1 N HCl, 10 μl/1.0 g sample.
II   contains 0.1 N HCl, 25 μl/1.0 g sample.
III contains 0.1 N HCl, 50 μl/1.0 g sample.
Condition: Temperature 70°C.

Table 5 — Effect of other alcohols on gelation process

Alcohol	Gelation time (hours:min)
Ethyl	1:00
Butyl	25:00
Pentyl	22:00
Hexyl	20:00
Heptyl	21:00
Octyl	20:00

Sample: TEOS 43%, alcohol 40%, water 8.5%, glycerol 8.5%.
Conditions: Temperature 70°C. Catalyst 0.1 N HCl, 10 μl/1.0 g sample.

ture conditions. Other additives such as glycerol affect the rate of gelation and the characteristics of the resulting gels. In these systems, ethanol and glycerol appear to play unique roles in the gelation process compared with other alcohols and polyhydric glycols. Overall, silica gels formed from organic silicates appear to be versatile systems with potential applications to the pharmaceutical industry. These systems have the capability to be modified and moulded to the specific needs of a desired drug delivery system.

REFERENCES

[1] M. Yamane, S. Aso, S. Okano and T. Sakaino, *J. Mater. Sci.*, **14**, 607 (1979).
[2] B. Yoldas, *J. Mater. Sci.*, **14**, 1843 (1979).
[3] K. Unger, H. Rupprecht, B. Valentin and W. Kircher, *Drug Dev. and Ind. Pharm.*, **9**(182), 69–91 (1983).
[4] K. D. Keefer, *Materials Research Society Symposium Proceedings*, Vol. 32, Elsevier Science Publishing Co., p. 15 (1984).
[5] L. C. Klein and G. J. Garvey, *Materials Research Society Symposium Proceedings*, Vol. 32, Elsevier Publishing Co., p. 33 (1984).
[6] R. A. Assink and B. D. Kay, *Materials Research Society Symposium Proceedings*, Vol. 32, Elsevier Science Publishing Co., (1984).
[7] C. J. Brinker, K. D. Keefer, D. W. Schaefer and C. S. Ashley, *J. Non-Cryst. Solids*, **48**, 47–64 (1982).
[8] R. A. Assink, B. D. Kay, C. S. Ashley, C. J. Brinker and K. D. Keefer, *J. Non-Cryst. Solids*, **63**, 45–59 (1984).
[9] R. Aelion, A. Loebel and F. Erich, *J. Am. Chem. Soc.*, **72**, 5705 (1950).

6

Microstructural changes during the storage of systems containing cetostearyl alcohol/polyoxyethylene alkyl ether surfactants

G. M. Eccleston and **L. Beattie**
Department of Pharmacy, School of Pharmacy and Pharmacology,
University of Strathclyde, Glasgow G1 1XW, UK

SUMMARY

Non-ionic emulsifying wax/water ternary systems composed of water, ceto-stearyl alcohol and non-ionic polyoxyethylene alkyl ether surfactants $(R=-(OCH_2CH_2)_A OH)$ with polyoxyethylene (POE) chain lengths, A, varying from 10–30 and R = cetostearyl were examined as they aged for several weeks. The techniques employed included rheological (Ferranti-Shirley cone and plate viscometer), microscopial (brightfield and between crossed polars), thermal (thermogravimetry and DSC) and ultra-centrifugation.

The rheological properties of the samples were complex. They confirmed, however, that all ternary systems increased in consistency on storage. For each ternary system apparent viscosities (η_{app}) increased as the samples aged. In addition, ternary systems prepared with surfactants with long POE chains were generally of a higher consistency then similar ternary systems containing shorter POE chains.

Each ternary system was considered to be composed of crystalline and gel (L_β) phases dispersed in bulk (free) water. The overall consistency of each system was related to the swelling ability and the relative amounts of gel phase present; this in turn depended on the POE chain length of the surfactant. The structural changes on storage were due to the formation of additional gel phase. This occurred because hydration of POE chains to form gel phase was limited at the high temperature of manufacture. On storage at lower temperature (25°C) the increased solubility of the POE chains allowed additional gel phase to form. However, this now occurred relatively slowly because of the crystalline nature of the hydrocarbon chains. Microscopical observations support this theory, for the timescale of observed interaction correlated well with the consistency and 'free' water changes on storage.

INTRODUCTION

Many dermatological emulsions are formulated using mixed emulsifiers of the surfactant/fatty alcohol type (emulsifying waxes). The surfactants may be ionic or non-ionic, although in general non-ionics are preferred, because they are less irritant to the skin and exhibit fewer incompatibilities with charged drugs and excipients than the ionics. Microstructural differences between ionic and non-ionic preparations are not always recognized. However, oil-in-water creams stabilized by such mixed emulsifiers are not simple two-phase oil-and-water emulsions, but multicomponent systems containing additional aqueous (e.g. lamellar liquid crystalline or gel) phases. These additional phases form when emulsifier, in excess of that necessary to form a monomolecular film at the oil droplet/water interface, interacts with water. The phase behaviour of a variety of ionic and non-ionic mixed emulsifier/water systems, and their relevance to cream microstructures have been the subject of recent reviews [1–3].

A major disadvantage of using non-ionic emulsifying waxes is that the resultant oil-and-water creams and lotions often gel-up after manufacture. This may result in a product which has unpredictable properties on storage and becomes so thick that it is unacceptable cosmetically or that drug bioavailability is altered. Rheological investigations into structural build-up showed that whereas ionic lotions and creams reached their normal semi-solid consistencies within a few hours of preparation, the consistencies of systems prepared with non-ionic emulsifying waxes increase considerably on extended storage [4–6]. Moreover, analysis of viscoelastic data clearly indicated that both the mechanism by which non-ionic and ionic preparations form and their final microstructures differ considerably [4,7].

The present chapter reports an investigation into such structural changes on storage, and is part of an overall investigation into the microstructures of complex pharmaceutical emulsions and the influence of drugs on them. For this work ternary systems, formed by mixing similar concentrations of mixed emulsifier in water to those used in commercial creams, were examined. Such ternary systems have been shown to be suitable models to study the structures of emulsion continuous phases [1,2]. The systems were prepared with a series of surfactants of increasing HLB number with polyoxyethylene chain lengths varying from 10–30.

MATERIALS AND METHODS
Materials
Water was double distilled and de-ionized. Cetostearyl alcohol BP (Evans, UK) and non-ionic surfactants of the polyoxyethylene alkyl ether type

$$(CH_3(CH_2)_XCH_2(OCH_2CH_2)_AOH$$

where X = 14 or 16 and A varied from 10 to 30 (Texofor A series, A.B.M. Chemicals, UK) were used as received. In the text individual surfactants are abbreviated as A10, A14, A18, A30 and A1P where the numbers denote the ethylene oxide chain length and A1P represents Cetomacrogol 1000 BPC (A = 20–24).

Preparation of ternary systems

Ternary systems were prepared according to the formulae in Table 1 by a

Table 1 — Composition of ternary systems (g)

	T,A10	T,A14	T,A18	T,A1P	T,A30
Surfactant*	3.6	4.6	5.5	6.4	8.2
C/S Alcohol	25.6	25.6	25.6	25.6	25.6
Water	300.0	300.0	300.0	300.0	300.0

* For each ternary system T, AX, X represents the surfactant polyoxyethylene chain length.

standardized procedure that involved melting the cetostearyl alcohol and surfactant together and adding water (which has been previously boiled to remove air) at approximately the same temperature (80°C), then cooling slowly while mixing with a Silverson homogenizer. The homogenizer speed was controlled throughout to avoid incorporation of air.

The molar ratios of each polyoxyethylene (POE) alkyl ether surfactant to cetostearyl alcohol (1:25) and the total concentration of each mixed emulsifier in water (10%) were chosen because with Cetomacrogol 1000 this molar ratio and concentration produces systems of the soft semisolid consistency used commercially. Samples were stored at 25°C.

Microscopy

Each ternary system was examined using the Polyvar microscope (Rheichart-Jung, Austria) in brightfield and between crossed polars. The systems were examined immediately after preparation and at frequent intervals over a one month storage period.

Rheology

Rheological experiments were performed at 25°C using a Ferranti-Shirley cone and plate viscometer in automatic mode with a sweep time of 600. The maximum shear rate was 1684 sec^{-1} and the resultant flow curves were displayed on an X–Y plotter. Samples were tested immediately after preparation and frequently over one month's storage.

Thermogravimetric analysis

The ratio of free and interlamellarly bound water was determined as systems aged using the thermogravimetric method described by De Vringer et al. [8]. This involves recording the weight loss at 2°C/minute (Stanton-Redcroft TG

750, UK) when about 4 mg of each ternary system was heated from ambient temperature to approximately 80°C (i.e. when no further weight loss was registered).

Ultracentrifugation
Samples were ultracentrifuged (MSE Superspeed 75, MSE, UK) at 25°C for times ranging from three to twenty hours at 130 000 g and the quantity of free water determined by weighing the water that separated.

Differential Scanning Calorimetry (DSC)
Preliminary DSC experiments between ambient and +100°C were performed on systems aged for about two months using the Mettler DSC 30 system (Mettler, Switzerland).

RESULTS

Appearance of systems
Sample T,A10 was a white, mobile lotion immediately after preparation and although some thickening was visible it remained mobile on storage. All other samples were semi-solids.

Microscopy
Representative photomicrographs of freshly prepared systems are shown in Fig. 1. In ordinary light, all ternary systems contained large masses of partially interacted emulsifying wax in addition to many smaller particles. The smaller particles which appeared as distorted Maltese crosses in polarized light, were present in fresh and aged systems. The partially interacted emulsifying wax was most prominent in T,A10, where large (often greater than 50 μm) dense masses of material with ciliated structures radiating from them, were apparent (Fig. 1(a)). These unreacted masses were smaller in ternary systems prepared with surfactants of longer POE chain lengths. For example, there were large numbers of particle sizes of up to 40 μm in system T,A14, but most were less than 25 μm in system T,A1P.

On extended storage, further interaction occurred and these structures had either disappeared altogether as in high POE systems, or had changed and reduced in size (low POE number system). In those masses remaining, they were mainly orientated into 'onion ring' structures rather than cilia and surrounded the central mass (cf. Figs 1(a), (b) and (c)).

Rheology
The flow curves obtained for all the samples were complex. Representative plots are shown in Fig. 2. Immediately after preparation samples T,A10 and T,A14 showed clockwise hysteresis loops and sometimes the up and down curves crossed over, implying that the shearing cycle itself causes some structural build-up. In aged samples, the flow curves reverted to the more usual anticlockwise hysteresis loops. The flow curves for the other systems (T,A18; T,A1P; T,A30) also changed after storage.

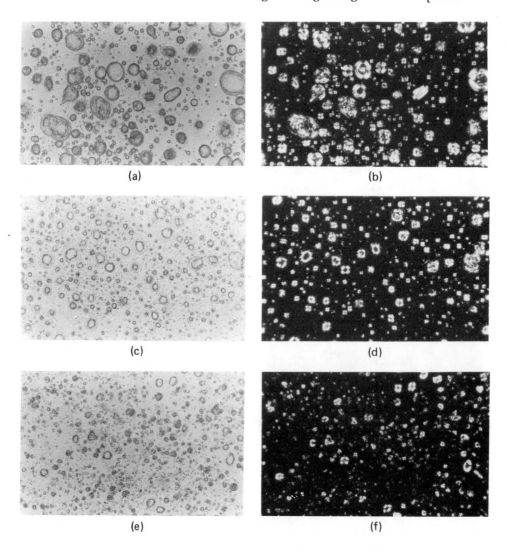

Fig. 1 — Representative photomicrographs of freshly prepared ternary systems in
brightfield and between crossed polars. (a) and (b) = T,A10; (c) and (d) = T,A14;
(e) and (f) = T,A1P.

All ternary systems showed increases in apparent viscosities on storage
but at different rates and to different extents (Fig. 3). For clarity, apparent
viscosities for initial and one month systems are shown in Table 2.

Systems prepared with shorter POE chain length surfactants are generally of a lower consistency, and show less structural build-up than those
containing longer POE chain lengths (cf. Table 2, Figs 2 and 3). It was noted
that although T,A30 was a highly structured semisolid, showing changes on
storage, its apparent viscosities were not as high as those expected from the

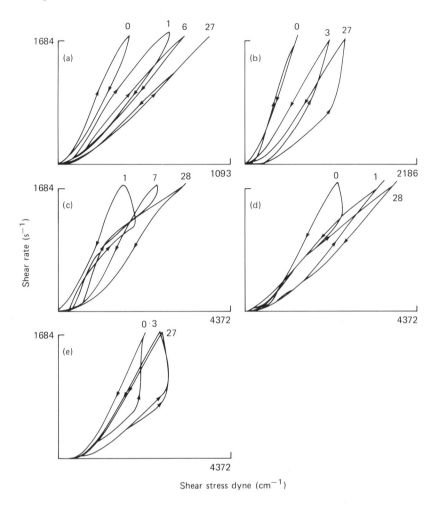

Fig. 2 — Ferranti-Shirley cone and plate viscometer. Representative flow curves for ternary systems (a) T,A10; (b) T,A14; (c) T,A18; (d) T,A1P and (e) T,A30, aged for the stated times (days).

general trend of increasing apparent viscosity increase with increasing POE chain length and its final consistency was lower than ternary systems T,A18 and T,A1P.

Ultracentrifugation

All the ternary systems separated into two layers after centrifugation. The top layer was thick, white semisolid and was composed mainly of distorted spherulites and crystalline material; the crystal masses appeared to have interacted further during centrifugation. The percentage of free water was calculated from the weight of water that separated as the bottom layer. Results obtained were erratic and are discussed later.

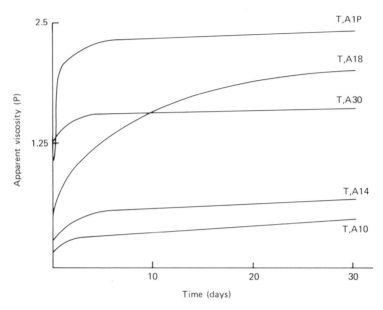

Fig. 3 — The variation of apparent viscosity at the loop apex, η_{app} (Poise), for each ternary system with storage time (days).

Table 2 — Apparent viscosities at the loop apex, η_{app} (Poise) immediately after preparation and after one month's storage

	T,A10	T,A14	T,A18	T,A1P	T,A30
0 hours	0.30	0.39	0.74	1.02	1.36
1 month	0.62	0.80	1.93	2.40	1.61

Thermogravimetric analysis

Figure 4 shows typical thermogravimetric curves for T,A30. Similar data were obtained for the other ternary systems throughout the storage cycle. In each ternary system there were two inflexions in the weight loss curve; the first peaking at 43°C and ending at 46–48°C and the second peaking at 55°C and ending at 62–63°C. In general, free water decreased both as samples aged and as the number of POE groups in the surfactant increased (Fig. 5), although values were again rather erratic.

Differential scanning calorimetry

DSC thermograms for aged systems were obtained. In all systems a broad endotherm starting about 50°C and peaking at 60°C was obtained (Fig. 6). The enthalpies were all approximately 11 J/g. This represented the melting enthalpies of the hydrocarbon chains of the mixed emulsifer.

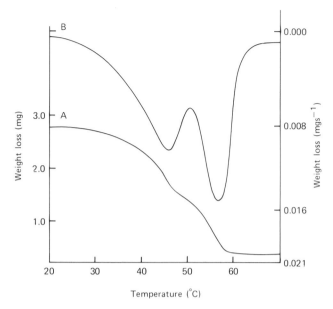

Fig. 4 — Typical thermogravimetric, A (mg) and differential thermogravimetric, B (mg s^{-1}) curves showing the stages of water loss (T,A30).

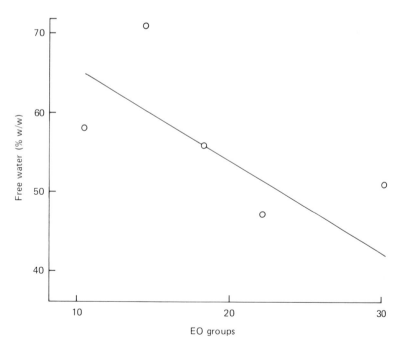

Fig. 5 — Variation of % free water (w/w) with the number of surfactant ethylene oxide groups for ternary systems aged for one month.

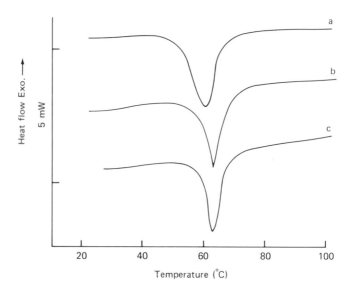

Fig. 6 — DSC data for ternary systems (a) T,A10; (b) T, A14 and (c) T,A1P, aged for two months.

DISCUSSION

Each ternary system is a multiphase system composed of hydrated crystalline cetostearyl alcohol and gel (L_β) phase dispersed in 'free' water. The gel phase consists essentially of crystalline hydrocarbon bilayers of alcohol and surfactant, separated by aqueous layers containing hydrated polyoxyethylene groups of the surfactant [2,9,10]. Microscopically, this phase is visible as large (often several μm, Fig. 1) multilamellar vesicles which show rather distorted extinction crosses in polarized light. Although fatty alcohol alone can only exhibit limited swelling to form crystalline hydrates, fatty alcohol/surfactant gel phases can swell to a much greater amount [2,3].

Structural changes in each sample were represented by apparent viscosity values (η_{app}) calculated at the apex of each hysteresis loop. Although such values should be treated with caution as they are not fundamental rheological parameters, they have been shown in the past to be useful guides of consistency in closely related systems, as long as they are also correlated with visual observation of flow curve changes. The rheological data confirmed that all ternary systems increased in consistency on storage and that the extent and time scale of these increases were related to the number of POE groups present in the surfactant. The structural changes were usually accompanied by reductions in the amount of free water. In addition, systems containing surfactants of high POE number contained less free water and were thicker than those containing shorter POE chains.

The techniques (ultracentrifugation and thermogravimetric) used to investigate the relative amounts of free and 'bound' water in each ternary system were not satisfactory. Although thermogravimetric results appeared to somewhat correlate with rheological data, in that systems of high consistency generally contained less free water, ultracentrifugation data were completely erratic, and no discernible trends were observed. Similar inconsistencies were observed by Rowe and Bray [11] in ultracentrifugation results for ionic emulsions. Water evaporation during preparation of the systems does not completely explain the grossly erratic results, nor does the fact that the consistency of each system will itself be increasing as water separates during centrifugation. It is possible that with these systems the strong forces experienced during centrifugation cause additional structural changes. Microscopial examinations of the system both before and after centrifugation implied that crystalline masses had further interacted. The inconsistencies ion thermogravimetric data were due to the fact that evaporation of these systems is a very complex phenomenon, possibly involving simultaneous dehydration of POE groups as well as evaporation of bulk water.

When these results are correlated with microscopical examinations, they imply firstly, that the overall consistency of each ternary system is related to the swelling ability and the amount of gel phase present, and secondly that the amount of gel phase relative to the other phases depends on the polyoxyethylene chain length of the surfactant.

Each ternary system was prepared by mixing molten alcohol and surfactant with water at a high temperature, and then cooling while still mixing, to the storage and testing temperature (25°C). A very complex phase situation is envisaged during this preparation procedure because hydration of the polyoxyethylene chains although limited at the high temperature, is continually increasing as the systems cool to the storage temperature. Above the hydrocarbon chain melting temperatures, mixed lamellar liquid crystalline and micellar phases are present as well as relatively large masses of molten alcohol and surfactant. In these masses the hydrocarbon chains of the surfactant are dispersed amongst those of the alcohol and the POE groups are present both at the surface and clustered within the masses.

As the systems cool and the POE regions become more soluble, water penetrates into the masses and, if the hydration forces are strong enough lamellar liquid crystals will separate. When the hydrocarbon chain crystallization temperature is reached (approx. 50°C — DSC data), the liquid crystals transform to a gel phase, and the partially hydrated emulsifying wax precipitates (Fig. 1). On storage, water continues to penetrate into the crystalline masses to further hydrate the POE regions, and additional gel phase forms. This occurs relatively slowly, because of the crystalline nature of the hydrocarbon chains causing water penetration and rearrangement into swollen gel bilayers to be extremely slow. As additional gel phase forms on storage, the amount of free water is reduced and the ternary systems thicken.

The tendency of the gel phase to separate from the crystalline masses and the thickness of the intralamellar water layers in this phase, will depend on the net repulsive forces caused by hydration. The nature of hydration forces have been discussed recently for polyoxyethylene alkyl ethers containing both short (<10) and long (up to 30) POE chains [12–15]. The so-called interlamellar or 'bound' water is considered to include all the arrangements of water molecules relative to the polyoxyethylene chains including hydrogen bonding, dipole interactions and water that is physically trapped both within and between the POE chains.

In ternary systems prepared with surfactants of short ethylene oxide chain length, especially T,A10, the hydrocarbon forces are not sufficient to force the hydrocarbon chains of the emulsifying wax crystals apart for significant quantities of additional gel phase to form on storage. Thus partially hydrated emulsifying wax masses are visible microscopically in both fresh and aged ternary systems T,A10 and T,A14. It was observed that the consistency of these systems had increased when sheared during rheological experiments. It is likely that the shearing forces mechanically disrupt the masses, exposing the surfactant chains to the water, with the formation of the additional gel phase.

As the POE chain length is increased from A10 to A30, hydration forces increase. Although only two molecules of water hydrate each ethylene oxide group by hydrogen bonding, long POE molecules may also trap additional water between the chains [16–19], thus additional gel phase separates from the masses. The thickness of the interlamellar layers will also be greater as POE chain length increases. Microscopically, the crystalline masses reduce in number and are smaller as POE chain length increases. The aged sample T,A30, although semi-solid, is of a lower consistency than expected. This may be because with very long POE chains, increased crowding now prohibits hydration of the surfactant so that the thickness of the interlamellar layers is smaller than expected.

CONCLUSIONS

Ternary systems composed of water, cetostearyl alcohol and non-ionic polyoxyethylene alkyl ether surfactants ($R-(OCH_2CH_2)_A OH$ with polyoxyethylene chain length A, varying from 10–30 and R = cetostearyl were examined as they aged using rheological microscopial, thermal and ultracentrifugation techniques. In general, ternary systems containing surfactants with longer POE chains were of a higher consistency and contained less free water than similar ternary systems prepared with shorter POE chains. In addition, each ternary system showed structural build-up on storage; as consistency increased free water decreased and microscopical changes were visible.

Each ternary system was found to be a multiphase system composed of hydrated crystalline cetosteary alcohol and α-crystalline gel (L_β) phase dispersed in 'free' water. The gel phase consisted essentially of crystalline hydrocarbon bilayers of alcohol and surfactant, separated by aqueous layers containing hydrated polyoxyethylene groups of the surfactant. This phase was identified microscopically by characteristic distorted extinction crosses in polarized light.

The overall consistency of each ternary system was related to the swelling ability and the amount of gel phase present; this in turn depended on the POE chain length of the surfactant. It was shown that the structural changes on ageing were due to the slow formation of additional gel phase on storage. As fresh gel phase forms, sequestration of free water occurs and the consistency of the ternary systems increase. The structural changes occur because hydration of POE chains is limited at the high temperatures of manufacture, but increases continually as the systems cool. On storage, the increased solubility of the POE chains causes additional gel phase to form. This occurs relatively slowly due to the slow rearrangements of crystalline hydrocarbon chains.

REFERENCES

[1] G. M. Eccleston, in *Chemistry of Materials used in Drug Delivery Systems. Critical Report on Applied Chemistry, Volume 6*. A. T. Florence (ed.), Blackwells, London, pp. 124 (1986).

[2] G. M. Eccleston, *Pharm. Internat.*, **7**, 63 (1986).

[3] G. M. Eccleston, *Cosmet. Toilet.*, **101**, 73 (1987).

[4] B. W. Barry and G. M. Saunders, *J. Colloid Interface Sci.*, **41**, 331 (1972).

[5] G. M. Eccleston, *J. Pharm. Pharmac.*, **29**, 157 (1977).

[6] G. M. Eccleston, *Int. J. Cosmetic Sci.*, **4**, 133 (1982).

[7] G. M. Eccleston, B. W. Barry and S. S. Davis, *J. Pharm. Sci.*, **62**, 1964 (1973).

[8] T. De Vringer, J. G. H. Joosten and H. E. Junginger, *Colloid and Polymer Sci.*, **264**, 691 (1986).

[9] T. De Vringer, J. G. H. Joosten and H. E. Junginger, *Colloid and Polymer Sci.*, **265**, 167 (1987).

[10] T. De Vringer, J. G. H. Joosten and H. E. Junginger, *Colloid and Polymer Sci.*, **265**, 448 (1987).

[11] R. C. Rowe and D. Bray, *J. Pharm. Pharmacol.*, **39**, 642 (1987).

[12] R. A. Mackay in *Nonionic Surfactants: Physical Chemistry*, M. Schick (ed.), Marcel Dekker, New York, Ch. 6 (1987).

[13] I. G. Lyle and G. J. T., Tiddy, *Chem. Phys. Lett.*, **124**, 432 (1986).

[14] M. Carvell, D. G. Hall, I. G. Lyle and G. J. T. Tiddy, *Faraday Discuss. Chem. Soc.*, **81**, 223 (1986).

[15] L. Marzall, *J. Dispersion Sci. and Tech.*, **2**, 443 (1981).

[16] P. H. Elworthy and C. B. MacFarlane, *J. Chem. Soc.*, **537** (1962).

[17] P. H. Elworthy, *J. Pharm. Pharmacol.*, **12**, 293 (1960).

[18] H. Schott, *J. Chem. and Eng. Data*, **11**, 417 (1966).

[19] D. I. D. El Eini, B. W. Barry and C. R. Rhodes, *J. Coll. Interface Sci.*, **54**, 348 (1975).

7

Structural stability of ophthalmic ointments containing soft paraffin

D. De Rudder, J. P. Remon
Laboratory of Pharmaceutical Technology, State University of Gent,
Harelbekestr. 72, B-9000 Gent, Belgium, and
P. Van Aerde
Alcon-Couvreur, Rijksweg 6, B-2670 Puurs, Belgium

INTRODUCTION

Soft paraffin (vaseline, petrolatum) is widely used in the formulation of pharmaceuticals and cosmetics. Soft paraffin is a plastic mass consisting of a mixture of solid and liquid saturated hydrocarbons (normal, iso and ring paraffins). The crystalline network of solid hydrocarbons encloses the liquid phase and immobilizes this fraction through adsorption, capillary action and molecular interactions [1].

Most of the drugs used in eye ointments are suspended in the excipient which contains mainly petrolatum. Several commercialized eye ointment formulations show structural breakdown and liquid separation (syneresis) leading to physical non-homogeneity of the ointment [2, 3]. During production it is necessary to mix the ingredients continually in order to maintain homogeneity during the cooling phase of the manufacturing process.

In this study the influence of the mixing process and the temperature treatment on a typical ointment base, is examined by oil number determination.

Basic characteristics of the petrolatum raw material such as 'final' viscosity melting enthalpy, X-ray diffraction and content of n-paraffins are correlated with oil numbers.

EXPERIMENTAL

Materials
All petrolatums and the lanolin oil used were of USP XXI grade.

Manufacturing methods

Composition of the ointment formulation — petrolatum/lanolin oil (97/3% w/w).

Laboratory scale production. Formulations were prepared in a Hobart planetary mixer (2 kg batch size). After melting (70°C), the mass was cooled to room temperature whilst stirring (100 r.p.m.).

Industrial scale production. Pilot batches (100 kg) were prepared in a Fryma VME 120 equipped with a homogenizer, a scraper and a stirrer. The homogenizer, used for drug dispersion, was not operated. The influence on the final consistency of the stirrer rate (1500, 1000 and 500 r.p.m.), of the scraper rate (10 and 2 r.p.m.) and of temperature treatment, was examined.

Analytical procedures

Differential scanning calorimetry. Several petrolatum samples and eye ointment formulations were submitted to a DSC analysis using a Perkin–Elmer DS calorimeter. Sample size was about 30 mg, the heating rate was $10°C\ min^{-1}$ at a range of 5 mcal/°C^{-1}. The melting enthalpy was calculated for all samples.

X-ray diffraction analysis. All samples analysed by DSC were submitted to X-ray diffraction analysis using a Philips X-ray diffraction apparatus (Philips P.A. 25, equipped with a copper anticathode 25 mA, 40 kV).

Viscosity determination. The 'final' viscosity was determined using a Haake RV 12 viscometer (N.V. spindle). The samples were heated to 55°C in the cup, cooled to room temperature and the 'final' viscosity was determined at room temperature (22°C) after 24 h.
   'Final' viscosity is defined as the minimum viscosity recorded at a constant shear of 2 r.p.m.

Oil number determination. 3 g vaseline or vaseline–lanoline oil blends were evenly spread on a Whatman paper no. 1 (12 cm×6 cm) over 5 cm×6 cm area. The strips of filter paper were supported vertically at room temperature and the height of ascent of oil measured after 24 h. The height of ascent expressed in millimetres is defined as the oil number. Oil numbers of experimental batches were determined within 24 h after production [4].

Determination of n-paraffin content in petrolatum samples. The method described by Presting and Boenke [5] was used. The experiments were performed on 10 g of the samples.

Production specifications. All batches were stirred and scraped until the temperatures of 50°, 40° or 30°C had been reached.
   Beyond this temperature batches were cooled to room temperature with and without scrapers in motion.

RESULTS AND DISCUSSION

Influence of processing parameters on the oil number
Figure 1 shows the influence of processing parameters, performed on

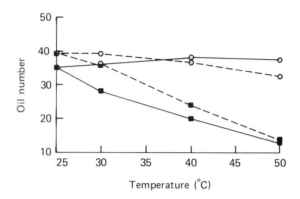

Fig. 1 — Oil numbers (of industrial batches) as a function of temperature at which stirring and/or scraping is stopped. The scraper rotational speed was kept constant at 10 r.p.m. The value on the X-axis indicates the temperature when stirring was stopped (+) or when both stirring and scraping were stopped (*). Two different speeds were selected for the stirrer: 500 r.p.m. (———); 1000 r.p.m. (···).

petrolatum 1–lanolin oil mixtures (97–3% w/w). The oil number is plotted versus the temperature at which stirring and/or scraping is stopped. The lowest oil number was obtained when both stirring and scraping were stopped at 50°C. The oil number increased progressively as the mechanical shear was applied up to the lowest temperatures. All batches produced while scraping was continued until room temperature, showed a high oil number, independent of the temperature at which stirring was stopped. It is obvious that scraping at lower temperatures, independent of stirring, has a dramatic influence on the oil number. Two levels of the scraper rotational speed were studied. The lower speed (2 r.p.m.) induced a distinct higher oil number than the higher one (10 r.p.m.) (Fig.2). Batches with an oil number over 25 showed visual syneresis after one week. Oil number values obtained from laboratory scale experiments were similar to those of the industrial batch productions indicating that scaling had no influence on the oil number.

Because shear induced syneresis could be attributed to a difference in the microcrystalline structure of the petrolatum, DSC and X-ray analysis were performed on two samples: an industrial batch with a low (A) and one with a high oil number (B). As can be seen from Table 1, the melting enthalpy of Batch A is approximately equal to Batch B.

This could indicate that the extent of microcrystalline structure formed during cooling is independent of the oil number and that chemical composition of the ointment rather then processing parameters may influence the

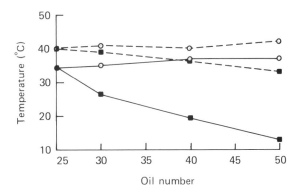

Fig. 2 — Oil numbers (of industrial batches) as a function of temperature at which stirring and/or scraping is stopped. The stirrer rotational speed was kept at 500 r.p.m. The value on the *X*-axis indicates the temperature when stirring was stopped (○) or when both stirring and scraping were stopped (■). Two different speeds were selected for the scraper: 10 r.p.m. (———), 2 r.p.m. (— — —).

Table 1 — Melting enthalpy and oil number for petrolatum–lanolin oil blends

	Melting enthalpy $(mcal/g^{-1})$	Oil number (mm)
Petrolatum–lanolin oil blend (97/3) (Batch A)	910	20
Petrolatum 1–lanolin oil blend (97/3) (Batch B)	981	40
Petrolatum–lanolin oil blend (97/3)	1317	19

bleeding tendency. These findings were confirmed by X-ray diffraction analysis. The low oil number of Batch A increased with time and reached the level of Batch B after 5 weeks.

Table 2 shows the relation between 'final' viscosity, oil number and *n*-paraffin content of commercial grade petrolatums.

A low oil number is related to a high 'final' viscosity, a hign *n*-paraffin content and a high melting enthalpy. As can be seen from Table 1, petrolatum 1, with a relative high oil number of 15, yielded a petrolatum–lanolin blend with a very high oil number of 40 while petrolatum 2 with an oil number of 5 produced an ointment with an oil number of only 19.

Table 2 — Oil number, 'final' viscosity and amount of n-paraffin for pure petrolatums

	Oil number (mm)	Melting enthalpy (mcal/g)	Final viscosity (mPa s)	Amount n-paraffin (gw/w)
Petrolatum 1	15	750	350	16.8
Petrolatum 2	5	1 225	10 653	40.6
Petrolatum 3	0	1 509	9 870	46.1

This may confirm that the chemical composition (content of n-paraffin) is the main factor influencing the physical stability of eye ointments on petrolatum basis.

CONCLUSION

Mechanical shear has a deleterious effect on the physical stability of petrolatum. The oil number determination may be a useful tool for the optimization of a production process and the prediction of physical ability of petrolatum ointments. Problems related to the syneresis of these ointments are basically dependent on the 'quality' of the petrolatum raw material.

Experimental production proved that with an oil number of pure petrolatum up to a value of 5, no problems of syneresis are encountered, even after application of mechanical shear. DSC and 'final' viscosity may give supplementary information for the selection of an appropriate petrolatum.

REFERENCES

[1] B. W. Barry and A. J. Grace, *Journal of Texture Studies*, **2**, 259 (1971).
[2] R. Cheng-Chyi Fu and D. M. Lidgate, *J. Pharm. Sci.*, **74**, 290 (1985).
[3] A. R. Longworth and J. D. French, *J. Pharm. Pharmacol.*, **21**, Suppl. 1S–5S (1969).
[4] H. J. Van der Pol, *Pharm. Weekbl.*, **9**, 3 (1960).
[5] W. Presting and R. Boenke, *Die Pharmazie*, **9**, 562 (1954).

8

The use of oscillatory rheological techniques to quantify the flow behaviour of polyelectrolyte systems

K. G. Hutchison, A. Li Wan Po and **R. A. Allison**
Department of Pharmaceutical Sciences, University of Aston in
Birmingham, Gosta Green, Birmingham B4 7ET, UK

INTRODUCTION

Rheological data is necessary to quantify various aspects of physical stability such as the prevention of sedimentation and ease of redispersion of a suspension, or prevention of coagulation and ease of extrusion from a tube for a cream product. Sedimentation rates in disperse systems are related to the viscosity measured at very low shear rates [1] but in some instances, it is the solid-like behaviour which prevents sedimentation [2]. Oscillatory shear methods provide a convenient way of determining both viscous and elastic components of a material independently [3,4].

In this study, oscillatory shear rheological techniques are used to demonstrate the application of fundamental data to flow problems in pharmaceutical formulation. Several polymeric solutions, dispersions and gels containing xanthan gum, carbopol and alginate are used to explain how oscillatory shear data is obtained and interpreted. The effects of processing on rheological profiles are demonstrated and comparisons with data obtained by traditional continuous shear techniques are made. Examples of oscillatory measurements of proprietary pharmaceutical suspensions are given.

EXPERIMENTAL

The instrument used was a Weissenberg rheogoniometer, model R16 with parallel 7.5 cm plate geometry. Measurements of amplitude ratio and phase lag were used to calculate the dynamic viscosity η' and storage modulus G'.

The instrument was used in a constant 20°C temperature laboratory. The gap between the plates was set to 0.508 mm throughout. Calibration of the gap setting, torsion head and oscillation displacement transducers was carried out using a micrometer.

To check the oscillatory function of the rheogoniometer, tests were carried out with the Newtonian liquids, silicone fluid 100 cs and liquid paraffin BP to obtain curves of amplitude ratio v and phase lag C against frequency. In accordance with theory, $v=1$ and $C=0$ at the reonant frequency of the instrument [5], that is $f=4$ Hz for a torsion bar with a constant $K_t=104$ dyne cm μm^{-1}. In addition, a viscoelastic sample of carbopol 941, 1.0% w/w was tested and found to give good agreement with similar experiments carried out by Barry and Meyer [6].

Repeated testing of several viscoelastic samples showed that G' and η' could be determined to within a precision of $\pm 5\%$. However, at low phase angles, small errors in C lead to large errors in η' due to the presence of a sine term in the equation used to calculate η' [7]. Also, at values of the amplitude ratio approaching 1.0, small errors in v lead to large errors in G'. Both of these effects are quantified and it is shown that significant errors are introduced when $C\neq 0$, $C<15°$, $v>0.96$.

RESULTS AND DISCUSSION

Xanthan gum

The oscillatory shear behaviour of a series of xanthan gum 0.4–4.0% w/w dispersions are given in terms of their $\eta'(\omega)$ and $G'(\omega)$ curves. As the polymer concentratrion is increased, a reduction in the slope of the G' line reflects the increase in solid-like behaviour and at higher frequencies, there is a tendency for the G' line to plateau at perhaps 10^2–10^3 rad s^{-1}. In the same frequency range, the slopes of the $\eta'(\omega)$ curves remain virtually unchanged. This change in the relative solid- and liquid-like behaviour can be summarized by plotting the ratio η'/G' which is the loss tangent, tan δ. This illustrated that although both G' and η' increase with xanthan gum concentration, the G' component rises more rapidly.

The properties of a dispersion of xanthan gum can be significantly affected by admixture with another polymer. The addition of sodium alginate was found to drastically reduce both the elastic and viscous components. The data for sodium alginate 0–8.0% w/w added to xanthan gum 2.0% w/w dispersions show that G' is much more affected than η'. This could be particularly important if the physical stability of a formulation is dependent upon the elastic component. The reason for alginate having such a drastic effect on xanthan gum structure is speculative. Every alternate side-chain to the main xanthan cellulose backbone has an attached pyruvate unit which is thought to be responsible for hydrogen bonding to adjacent side-chains. It is this interaction which imparts the gel-like behaviour.

It is further hypothesized that the carboxyl groups of the guluronic and mannuronic acid residues of the alginate could also interact by hydrogen bonding to the xanthan side-chains. This would reduce the total number of cross-linkages because alginate is unable to cross-link in the absence of divalent metal ions.

Carbopol

Similar experiments were carried out using Carbopol 934P dispersions which had been gelled by neutralization with sodium hydroxide. In accordance with the gel-like nature of carbopol, viscous behaviour was only observed at low concentrations of 0.2% w/w. At higher concentrations almost purely elastic behaviour was characterized by only small changes in elastic modulus G' with frequency. On addition of sodium alginate in concentrations up to 5.0% w/w to a carbopol 0.8% w/w gel, there was a drastic reduction in the elastic component and the systems became free-flowing. This is illustrated by the appearance of a series of $\eta'(\omega)$ curves. By taking the G' and η' at one frequency only, and plotting against added alginated concentration, the greater reduction in elasticity compared to viscosity can be demonstrated. In this instance, it is likely to be the ionic nature of alginate which breaks down carbopol structure, since the latter is known to be sensitive to the addition of electrolyte.

Calcium alginate

Oscillatory shear testing is particularly suited to gel samples which are of a weak or brittle nature since the net deformation during testing is negligible. Calcium alginate gels were prepared by mixing a dispersion of calcium hydrogen phosphate in sodium alginate solution with a solution of glucono-δ-lactone. The gradual reduction in pH caused by hydrolysis of glucono-δ-lactose to gluconic acid allowed a gradual release of calcium ions into solution and the formation of a homogeneous gel [8]. Gels were formed into flat discs which were the correct dimensions to be placed between the parallel plates of the rheogoniometer.

Data for the elastic modulus obtained for an increasing concentration of alginate showed a marked tendency towards purely elastic behaviour at a concentration of approximately 3% w/v alginate when the calcium concentration was held constant at 50 mm0l. When the alginate concentration was maintained at 3% w/v, an increasing concentration of calcium ions showed a similar plateau of purely elastic behaviour. Measurable viscous behaviour was only recorded for gels containing 10 mmol calcium and even for this sample, the G' data showed little variation with frequency.

Experiments carried out to monitor the diffusion of ibuprofen through the calcium alginate gels showed that the diffusion coefficients in gels containing 70 mmol of calcium did not change significantly when the alginate concentration increased from 0.25 to 5.0% w/v. In addition, diffusion coefficients obtained were similar to the free diffusion coefficient of ibuprofen in water. Combined with the rheological data, it is likely that although increasing alginate concentration increased the elastic modulus, the pore size within the gel matrix was insufficient to impede the diffusion of the ibuprofen molecule.

Shearing effects
The effects of shearing of polymer mixes of xanthan and alginate, and carbopol and alginate were investigated. Mixes were prepared using paddle stirrers but then subjected to high shear by means of a Silverson AXR homogenizer. Mixes containing xanthan and alginate showed marked increases in dynamic viscosity η' with increasing time, but the elastic modulus G' increased by an even greater proportion. However, more prolonged shearing resulted in reduced η' and G' values which indicated irreversible shear breakdown.

Comparison of oscillatory and continuous shear data
The addition of alginate to carbopol gels has been shown to have characteristic effects on η' and G'. Although this can yield helpful quantitative information, it would be useful to known whether continuous shear data can provide qualitatively comparable results. A Rheomat 30 viscometer was used to obtain shear stress versus shear rate rheograms over a shear rate range 53.6 to 3950 s^{-1}. Empirical equations were applied, and using non-linear regression analysis [9], the best fit was obtained using the Shangraw equation [10]:

$$\tau = f + \eta_\alpha \dot{\gamma} - b_v \exp^{-a\dot{\gamma}}$$

where τ is the shear stress, $f - b_v$ is the yield stress, η_α is the limiting high shear viscosity, $\dot{\gamma}$ is the shear rate and a is the empirical constant.

It was shown that plots of η_α or f against alginate concentration were quantitatively and qualitatively different to η' and G' data obtained using oscillatory shear techniques. In addition, application of the Cox–Merz rule [11] which correlates frequency of oscillation with shear rate of continuous shear testing, was unable to correlate the data obtained by the two different methods.

Proprietary preparations
A series of proprietary pharmaceutical suspensions were tested in oscillatory shear and found to display very widely varying behaviour. The storage of samples of some of these products for short periods at 50°C gave rise to significant changes in rheological behaviour.

CONCLUSIONS

The careful use of rheological data obtained from oscillatory shear testing can lead to an understanding of how rheological behaviour affects the performance and physical stability of liquid and semisolid formulations.

REFERENCES

[1] R. Buscall, J. W. Goodwin, R. H. Ottewill and Th. F. Tadros, *J. Coll. Interface Sci.*, **85**, 78–86 (1982).
[2] K. Strenge, and H. Sonntag, *Coll. Polym. Sci.*, **252**, 133–137 (1974).

[3] J. D. Ferry, *Viscoelastic Properties of Polymers*, J. Wiley, 3rd edn (1980).

[4] G. W. Scott-Blair *Elementary Rheology*, Academic Press (1969).

[5] K. Walters, *Rheometry*, Chapman & Hall, London (1975).

[6] B. W. Barry and M. C. Meyer, *Int. J. Pharm.*, **2**, 1–25 (1979).

[7] B. Warburton and S. S. Davis, *Rheol. Acta*, **8**, 205–214 (1969).

[8] J. R. Mitchell and J. M. V. Blanchard, *J. Texture Studies*, **7**, 219–234 (1976).

[9] C. M. Metzler, G. L. Elfing and A. J. McEwen, *A Users Manual for NONLIN and Associated Programmes*, Upjohn Co., Michigan (1974).

[10] R. Shangraw, W. Grim and A. M. Mattocks, *Trans. Soc. Rheol.*, **5**, 247–260 (1961).

[11] W. P. Cox and E. H. Merz, *J. Polymer Sci.*, **28** (118), 619–623 (1958).

9

Advantages of the use of very short and ultra-short HPLC columns for drug analysis in dissolution testing

Peter Timmins
Pharmaceutical Sciences Department, International Development
Laboratory, Squibb Pharmaceutical Products, Reeds Lane, Moreton,
Wirral, Merseyside L46 1QW, UK

SUMMARY

The advantage of short (3–5 cm long) or ultra-short (4 mm long) HPLC columns for drug analysis in dissolution testing are illustrated by reference to some example antihypertensive formulations. Advantages include:

(a) Selectivity, where interfering excipients or co-formulated drugs complicate UV spectrophotometric analysis.
(b) Time savings, compared with conventional HPLC columns (although where UV spectrophotometry is applicable no time advantages may be obtained with short column HPLC).
(c) Economy, as the columns are less expensive than conventional columns and there is reduced solvent consumption.
(d) Increased sensitivity compared with conventional columns. Low dose potent drugs with poor chromophores may be more readily quantified.
(e) Amenity to automation, including the use of laboratory robots.

These advantages would suggest the wide applicability to this mode of analysis in dissolution testing.

INTRODUCTION

In-vitro dissolution testing is an important tool in the development and quality control of solid dosage forms. Basically, the test consists of measuring the rate of release of drug from a solid dosage form into an aqueous environment under defined conditions. Samples of test solution are taken at one or more time points and the concentrations of dissolved drug or drugs are determined. In a typical test six tablets or capsules would be tested simultaneously.

Traditionally, UV spectrophotometry has been used to determine the amount of dissolved drug. However, modern potent drugs may be present in low doses and additionally have weak chromophores, making spectrophotometry difficult. A number of drugs may be co-formulated into a single dose unit to aid patient compliance. Such formulations may present problems in spectrophotometric analysis requiring measurement at multiple wavelengths with associated calculations, or the dedication of an expensive photodiode array spectrophotometry.

High performance liquid chromatography (HPLC) may provide an answer in selectivity and sensitivity to resolve the above-mentioned problems, but can be slow, with each sample analysis taking up to thirty minutes to complete. Such analysis times would mean that samples need to be deposited in a fraction collector for subsequent analysis, although Wurster et al. [1] have already described an automated dissolution system with direct introduction of samples into an HPLC system. This latter system is only applicable to analysis of samples from a single dissolution vessel in most instances. With conventional HPLC columns, analysis times are such that direct sampling from a number of vessels at time points separated by only a few minutes would not be possible.

To obtain the benefits of HPLC and reduce analysis time, very short (3–5 cm long) HPLC columns and 4 mm long guard columns have been used in this work as ultra-short analytical columns for the analysis of drug solutions during dissolution testing. There are some published reports in the use of very short columns in pharmaceutical analysis [2,3], but the only publication on the application to dissolution testing [3] highlights the speed of such techniques and their amenity to automation.

The present work demonstrates the advantages of short column HPLC when applied to some example antihypertensive formulations, where potent drugs with weak chromophores or combination formulations are involved. The further advantages and general applicability of this approach to drug analysis in dissolution testing are highlighted.

EXPERIMENTAL

Equipment
Dissolution tests were undertaken in a USP rotating basket apparatus having six test stations (Hanson 72 RL, Copley Instruments, Nottingham, UK, or Caleva, DT7, G.B. Caleva, Ascot, UK). Samples were taken manually into 10 ml plastic syringes or automatically employing an autosampler (Caleva 3-10, G.B. Caleva, Ascot, UK). Filtration was achieved using disposable filters (Gelman 25 mm Acrodisc, 0.45 μm pore size, Gelman Sciences, Northampton, UK, and porous polypropylene in-line filters, cat. no. 1504, Copley Instruments, Nottingham, UK, respectively).

Chromatography was undertaken employing a constant volume reciprocating pump (Altex 110A, Anachem, Luton, UK), a variable weavelength detector (Cecil CE212A, Talbot Instruments, Alderley Edge, UK), and an autoinjector (Talbot AS13, Talbot Instruments, Alderley Edge, UK). Chromatograms were recorded on a servoscribe 1S chart recorder (Brunner Instruments, Scarborough, UK).

Very short HPLC columns were packed with 3 μm C18 reversed-phase material (Perkin–Elmer, Beaconsfield, UK or Technicol, Stockport, UK). Ultra-short columns were 4 mm long C18 reversed phase-guard column cartridges held in a guard column holder (Waters Instruments, Harrow, UK), and were employed in place of the coventional analytical column.

Applications

Tablets containing 12.5 mg of the antihypertensive agent captopril (E. R. Squibb, Moreton, UK) were subjected to a dissolution test employing 1000 ml of 0.1 M hydrochloric acid in each vessel as dissolution medium. Chromatographic analysis was undertaken on a 3 cm long C18 reversed phase column and an eluting solvent consisting of methanol:water:85% phosphoric acid (380:620:0.4 v/v/v) was employed at a flow rate of 1.0 ml min^{-1}. The detector was set at 218 nm and 50 μl of sample injected via the autoinjector.

A development antihypertensive agent formulated as 10 mg of drug in capsules (E.R. Squibb, Moreton, UK) was subjected to a dissolution test employing 500 ml of 0.1 M hydrochloric acid as dissolution medium. Chromatographic analysis was undertaken on a 4 mm long C18 reversed phase-guard column used as an ultra-short analytical column. The solvent was methanol:phosphate buffer (pH 2.0) (3:7 v/v) delivered at 0.2 ml min^{-1}. The detector was set at 221 nm and 50 μl of sample injected.

A combination formulation containing 50 mg of captopril and 15 mg of the diuretic hydrochlorothiazide in a tablet (E. R. Squibb, Moreton, UK) was subjected to dissolution testing using the rotating basket method and employing 1000 ml of 0.1 M hydrochloric acid as dissolution medium. For simultaneous analysis of both drugs, HPLC on a 5 cm long reversed phase C18 column was employed, using methanol:0.5% aqueous phosphoric acid (20:80 v/v) at 1.0 ml min^{-1} as eluting solvent. Injection volume was 20 μl and the variable wavelength detector was set at 210 nm to obtain suitable peak height relationships, as the two drugs involved have very different chromophores.

RESULTS AND DISCUSSION

In-vitro dissolution testing of the antihypertensive drug captopril involves Ellmans reagent colorimetry of the thiol group for drug analysis. However, this approach requires preparation of a number of reagents, colour development and finally spectrophotometry. Hence, the method is time consuming, although automation of such methods is possible. Furthermore, the method is non-specific, as other thiol compounds, for example captopril hydrolysis products [4], would react with the reagent.

A specific HPLC method used in preformulation studies on captopril [4] can be used to separate and quantify captopril in dissolution media. By use of a 3 cm long column, rather than a 20 cm long column, total analysis time per time point sample was reduced to less than two minutes. A typical chromatogram is shown in Fig. 1. Compared with the 20 cm long column the

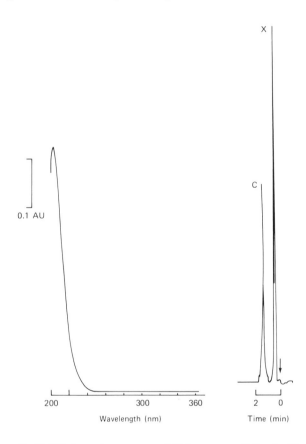

Fig. 1 — (Left) UV absorption spectrum of 12.5 mg captopril dissolved in 1000 ml of 0.1 N hydrochloric acid. (Right) Chromatogram of dissolution medium during dissolution test on 12.5 mg captopril tablet. C = captopril; X = excipients.

time to complete analysis of four time point samples from each of six dissolution vessels was reduced from around 4 hours to less than 1 hour. Table 1 indicates the total times required to complete analysis of four time points from each of six dissolution vessels by colorimetric and HPLC methods.

Because of the time savings, HPLC solvent consumption was also reduced. The shorter column length resulted in an approximately fivefold

Table 1 — Times to complete determination of captopril concentrate for four time point samples from each of six vessels during dissolution testing

	Colorimetry	HPLC (20 cm col.)	HPLC (30 cm col.)
Reagent or HPLC solvent preparation	2.5 h	0.3 h	0.3 h
Colour	0.3 h	—	—
Development analysis	0.3 h	4.2 h	0.9 h

increase in sensitivity. This latter advantage allowed for the quantitation of captopril from a 12.5 mg potency tablet formulation in 1000 ml of dissolution medium, in spite of the weak end absorption chromophore of captopril (Fig. 1).

With a second development antihypertensive agent separation of the active drug from capsule excipients could be achieved on a 4 mm long guard column (Fig. 2), which could be regarded as an ultra-short analytical column. In this case analysis is very rapid providing significant time savings, reduced solvent consumption and inexpensive columns when replacements are required. Such rapid analyses are suitable for on-line use, with a laboratory robot or a sampling value sequentially selecting form each dissolution vessel and a standard solution. Time between cycles would be short enough to permit dissolution profiling of even rapidly dissolving formulations in this way.

Combinations of the diuretic hydrochlorothiazide with captopril could be analysed in dissolution media by HPLC. Separation was on a very short reversed phase C18 column allowing simultaneous quantitation, saving considerable time over traditional individual colorimetric methods. With the colorimetric methods it may only be possible to analyse one or two batches of tablets manually, per day, whereas the HPLC method could theoretically allow for analysis of four or more lots. A typical chromatogram for the separation of captopril and hydrochlorothiazide in dissolution media on a 5 cm long column is shown in Fig. 3. The very short column methods provide for savings in time, solvent and expense compared with typical 25–30 cm columns previously used to analyse these components in intact tablets [5] and that are applicable to dissolution testing.

There are some problems with the use of HPLC to analyse samples of dissolution media. Acidic media such as 0.1 N hydrochloric acid can reduce column lifetime to just a few weeks. Fortunately such columns are less expensive than their conventional counterparts. In the examples given here a relatively inexpensive detector has been satisfactory, but for very rapid analysis it is desirable to use a more expensive detector with a short time constant to obtain optimal resolution of closely eluting peaks [2].

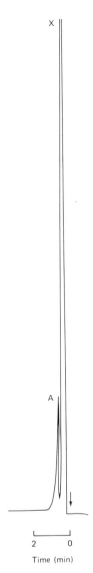

Fig. 2 — Chromatogram of dissolution medium during dissolution test on a development antihypertensive agent (A) using an ultra-short column. X = excipients.

Finally, although general applicability of this method is possible, the application to simple formulations where direct spectrophotometry is straightforward (e.g. high dose drugs with good chromophores), may lead to no advantages and tie up expensive HPLC equipment.

In summary, the advantages of very short or ultra-short HPLC columns in dissolution testing are:

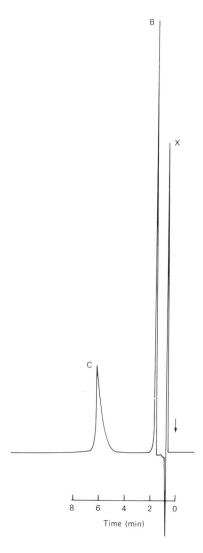

Fig. 3 — Chromatogram of dissolution medium during dissolution test on a tablet containing captopril and hydrochlorothiazide. C = Captopril; B = hydrochlorothiazide; X = excipients.

Selectivity, allowing separation of co-formulated drugs for simultaneous quantitation. Where reduced selectivity is acceptable, guard columns may be used as ultra-short columns to separate drug from excipients.

Time saving, as reduced analysis times compared with conventional HPLC columns are obtained.

Economy, as columns are less expensive than conventional columns and reduced analysis times lead to reduced solvent consumption.

Sensitivity is increased owing to the reduced column length, hence low dose potent drugs with weak chromophores may be more readily quantitated compared with conventional columns.

Amenable to automation. With the very short analysis times it is feasible that dissolution medium can be sampled directly into the chromatograph, either by selection and injection valves or via laboratory robots.

REFERENCES

[1] D. Wurster, W. Wargin and M. DeBaradinis, *J. Pharm. Sci.*, **70** (1981).
[2] J. C. Gfeller, R. Haas, J. M. Troendle and F. Erni, *J. Chromatog.*, **294**, 247 (1984).
[3] R. Soltero, J. Robinson and D. Adair, *J. Pharm. Sci.*, **73**, 799 (1984).
[4] P. Timmins, I. M. Jackson and Y. J. Wang, *Int. J. Pharmaceutics*, **11**, 329 (1982).
[5] J. Kirschbaum and S. Perlman, *J. Pharm. Sci.*, **73**, 686 (1984).

10

Dissolution of chlorpropamide tablets in a methanol–water binary solvent system

Alison Dodge and **Philip L. Gould**
Pharmaceutical Group, Product Research & Development Laboratories,
Cyanamid of Great Britain Limited, Gosport, Hampshire, UK

SUMMARY

The dissolution of 250 mg chlorpropamide tablets has been investigated in aqueous methanol co-solvent systems. Dissolution in the mixed solvent systems, despite sink conditions being obtained, was reduced over non-sink conditions in the pure aqueous system owing to impaired tablet disintegration. However, tablet disintegration was improved at low methanol volume fractions due to improved wetting and fluid flux into the tablet mass.

A dissolution system was devised using an appropriate amount and order of addition of methanol to the dissolution fluid.

INTRODUCTION

Dissolution of high dose relatively insoluble drugs such as chlorpropamide can be problematic owing to difficulties of maintaining the sink condition of the dissolution test. In such instances, where a readily accessible ionization centre to enhance solubility is not available, the formulator then considers adding a non-aqueous co-solvent such as an alcohol to the dissolution fluid. Poirier and others [1] have conducted studies on low dose chlrothalidone in an aqueous-ethanol co-solvent system and have pointed out that the nature of the co-solvent, and time of addition of the co-solvent to the dissolution fluid, can influence the resultant dissolution profile.

This work reports an investigation of a water–mathanol co-solvent dissolution test for tablets of this high dose hydrophobic drug chlorpropamide.

EXPERIMENTAL

Materials
Chlorpropamide tablets (250 mg Diabinese®) from Pfizer Ltd, Sandwich, UK. The chlorpropamide bulk used for the standards was to BP grade and obtained from Francis SpA, Italy. The methanol employed was AnalaR grade.

Methods
Drug solubility and determination of the sink condition
Chlorpropamide has a low solubility in water (0.27 mg/ml at 37°C) and therefore exceeds the sink condition, defined as 10% saturation, in the conventional USP paddle dissolution test. The amount of drug that can dissolve under sink conditions (900 ml) in a USP dissolution test is approximately 24 mg. Thus, dissolution of 250 mg tablets will require the addition of a co-solvent to the dissolution fluid to maintain sink conditions.

Solubilities of chlorpropamide were conducted at 37($\pm$1)°C by equilibrating excess drug with 10 ml of the binary aqueous methanol co-solvent system. Following equilibration, the solutions were filtered (Acrodisc, 0.2 μm) and diluted to a suitable concentration with methanol to allow spectrophotometric analysis at 230.9 nm.

Dissolution
Dissolution tests were conducted on a pre-calibrated dissolution bath (Caleva model 7ST, G.B. Caleva, Ascot, UK) according to the method in USP XXI using paddles at 50 r.p.m. The values reported are the mean of six determinations.

Disintegration
Tablet disintegrations were measured using the BP test using one tablet per tube. Each value reported is the mean of six determinations. The fluids employed were pure water and binary 10% v/v, 20% v/v, 40% v/v and 60% v/v methanol–water systems.

RESULTS AND DISCUSSIONS
Dissolution of the tablets under non-stick conditions in distilled water is shown in Fig. 1. As expected, dissolution is slow and incomplete with only 50% of the drug dissolved in 60 min. Measurement of the solubility of chlorpropamide at 37°C in an aqueous methanol system (Fig. 2) indicates that sink conditions are obtained with approximately 40% v/v methanol in the dissolution fluid. However, dissolution in the binary co-solvent system, even when sink conditions are maintained, leads to a more retarded dissolution profile (only 40% of chlorpropamide dissolving in 60 min (Fig. 1)) than in the pure aqueous fluid.

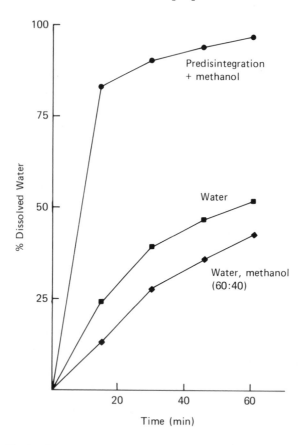

Fig. 1 — Dissolution of 250 mg chlorpropamide tablets in various fluids.

These dissolution results can be explained by the effect of methanol on the disintegration time of the tablets and is a result in accord with the work of Poirier and others [1], and also Guyot-Hermann and Ringard [2]. This was confirmed by measurement of the disintegration times of the chlorpropamide tablets at varying methanol levels in the aqueous fluid used for this disintegration test. The results (Fig. 3) show that, as expected, tablet disintegration in 40% methanol is some 20% longer than in pure water. The disintegration time is essentially doubled in 60% methanol.

Interestingly, and conversely to the previous work with low dose chlorthalidone [1], disintegration of chlorpropamide tablets in 20% methanol is some 20% faster than in pure water. Thus, in this tablet system, there appear to be two opposing forces governing tablet disintegration in the mixed solvent system. Addition of the co-solvent appears to prolong disintegration by hindering disintegrant swelling, but this is balanced against the improved wettability and resultant wicking of the disintegrating fluid into the tablet. This appears to occur with a fluid containing 30% v/v methanol which

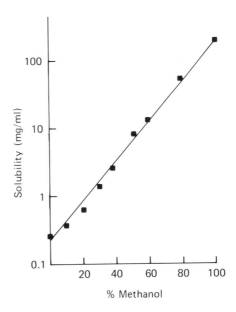

Fig. 2 — Solubility of chlorpropamide in binary water–methanol co-solvent system.

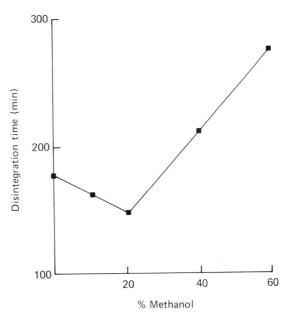

Fig. 3 — Disintegration times of 250 mg chlorpropamide tablets in binary methanol-
–water system.

possesses a surface tension of 44 mN m^{-1}. It is perhaps worthy of note that this balance of properties could be different in wet massed systems if the tablet contains intra- or extragranularly located disintegrant.

The balance of the disintegration phase in the mixed solvent, with the limitations from non-sink conditions in the tablet dissolution process was next examined by conducting studies using 20, 30, 40 and 60% aqueous-methanol systems. Dissolution of chlorpropamide from the tablets was found to be fastest with a fluid of 30% methanol (Fig. 4); the composition of

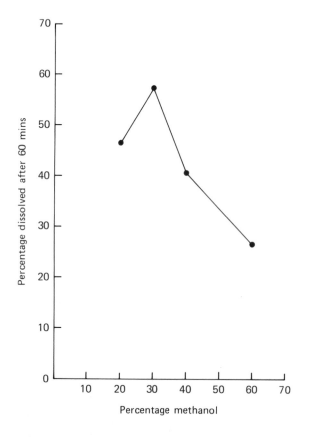

Fig. 4 — Percentage chlorpropamide dissolved in 60 minutes.

optimal tablet disintegration. However, even at 30% methanol, dissolution is relatively slow with only 58% drug dissolving in 60 minutes, owing to the methanol component being below that (40%) required for sink conditions.

Dissolution was next examined by allowing tablet disintegration within the aqueous component of fluid (540 ml) followed by addition of the methanol component after 10 min. A full dissolution profile from the tablets was obtained with over 90% of the drug released in 30 min (Fig. 1). Thus, allowing for unimpaired disintegration and maintaining the sink condition, full dissolution of the dosage forms can be demonstrated.

Conducting the same procedure with a 30% methanol system (non-sink) resulted, as before in incomplete dissolution (77% drug dissolved in 60 min) whereas the procedure using 60% methanol, produced an identical dissolution profile to that using 40% methanol (Table 1).

Table 1 — Percent dissolved from chlorpropamide tablets using a pre-disintegration technique with varying methanol levels in the binary solvent

% Methanol (time/min)	% Dissolved		
	30	40	60
15	38±9	75±5	77±2
30	66±2	90±3	96±3
45	74±1	94±3	99±3
60	77±1	96±2	100±4

However, there are a few artefacts of the solvent addition method that are worthy of note. In the first phase of the dissolution, during the mandatory aqueous disintegration phase, the hydrodynamics of the test are substantially altered by the reduced fluid volume. Following tablet disintegration, a further disruption in the solution hydrodynamics occurs owing to the addition of the non-aqueous phase. Perhaps, most importantly, following the second phase of solvent introduction, a temperature increase of 5°C occurs owing to exothermic heat of mixing of the two solvents. To investigate the above, a pre-disintegration dissolution test was conducted using water at 42°C as the added secondary phase. An increase in dissolution was indeed observed (62% versus 50% dissolved in 60 min), but the enhancement was significantly smaller than that produced with the co-solvent addition.

CONCLUSIONS

This study has investigated the influence of a binary co-solvent fluid on the disintegration phase within the dissolution process of a high dose solid dosage form of a relatively insoluble hydrophobic drug. Different tablet disintegration phenomena appear to apply depending on the level of the non-aqueous component of the mixed solvent system. However, despite tablet disintegration being improved at some solvent compositions, a phase of pre-disintegration of solid dosage forms should be incorporated in dissolution tests employing binary solvent mixtures.

REFERENCES

[1] H. Poirier, G. A. Lewis, M. J. Shott and H. N. E. Stevens, 'Problems with a pharmacopoeial dissolution test using a binary medium', *Drug Dev. Ind. Pharm.*, **9**, 442–452 (1983).

[2] A. M. Guyot-Hermann and J. Ringard, 'Disintegration mechanisms of tablets containing starches. Hypothesis about the particle–particle repulsive force', *Drug Dev. Ind. Pharm.*, **7**, 155–177 (1981).

11

pH measurements of suspensions

Geoffrey Lee, Douglas Dick, Eva Marie Vasquez and **Kimberly Werner**
Department of Pharmaceutics, College of Pharmacy, University of Illinois at Chicago, Illinois, USA

SUMMARY

Various pH measurements on silica suspensions have been made. The changes in pH of HCl/NaOH solutions caused by the addition of increasing amounts of dispersed phase were determined. These changes were pH dependent and could be as high as three pH units. The differences in measured pH between the silica suspensions and their supernatant liquids were also determined. These pH differences were due to the suspension effect, and were up to two pH units in magnitude. These results give an indication of the errors in pH which can be found when suspensions are not first centrifuged prior to determination of their pH.

INTRODUCTION

The stability of pharmaceutical suspensions is often greatly influenced by the presence of an electrostatic charge on the solid particles. In many cases, the magnitude of this surface charge is affected by the pH of the continuous phase. The measurement of the pH of suspensions is not, however, a straightforward matter. Measurement of the pH of the continuum before addition of the solid phase neglects the possibility of loss of continuum ions by adsorption on to the solid surface. Measurement of pH of the suspension itself may be liable to error as a result of the suspension effect.

The theoretical implications of both of these possible sources of error are well established in the field of colloid science, but receive less attention in pharmaceutical work. Many published studies of the properties of suspensions refer only vaguely to the methods used to measure pH. Indeed, there is little practical guide to the magnitude of the errors in pH to be expected from the two above-named effects. This work describes a systematic examination of pH measurement in a model suspension, namely that of the flame-hydrolysed silica Aerosil 200. From the results obtained, some general conclusions regarding the pH measurement of suspensions can be made. These are of relevance to the industrial pharmacist struggling to formulate any colloidal system.

EXPERIMENTAL

Solutions of pH 1 to 5 were prepared from HCl, and of pH 6 to 11 from NaOH. The pH of each solution (designated pH_b) was measured under nitrogen using a combination gel-filled eelctrode, as may be found in any industrial laboratory. Sols were then prepared by dispersing the Aerosil 200 powder in each pH-solution using ultrasonic radiation. The pH of each sol (designated pH_s) was then measured. Subsequently, each sol was centrifuged to remove the dispersed phase, and the pH of the supernatant measured (designated Ph_e).

Two parameters were calculated. First, the change in pH of the HCl or NaOH solution caused by the addition of the solid phase:

$$\Delta pH^{b-e} = pH_b - pH_e$$

Secondly the difference in pH between the sol itself and its supernatant liquid:

$$\Delta pH^{s-e} = pH_s - pH_e$$

The effects of three concentrations of solid phase on both ΔpH^{b-e} and ΔpH^{s-e} were determined, namely 0.1%, o.5% and 2.5% (all w/w).

RESULTS

All of the data are presented as plots of ΔpH^{s-e} or ΔpH^{b-e} versus pH_e. The 0.1% sols show small values for ΔpH^{s-e} (Fig. 1), changing from slightly negative at low pH_e to slightly positive at high pH_e.

This change is more pronounced with the 0.5% sols and clearly seen with the 2.5% sols. In this latter case, ΔpH^{s-e} becomes increasingly negative up to pH_e of about 6.5. Further increase in pH_e then reduces ΔpH^{s-e}, although values remain positive.

In contrast, the ΔpH^{b-e} values at all three solid concentrations are marginally negative up to pH_e of around 4 (Fig. 2), above which they become increasingly positive. The higher the solid concentration, the greater the value of ΔpH^{b-e}.

With the 2.5% sols, however, the ΔpH^{b-e} values show a plateau in the pH_e range 5 to 7, above which there is a slight decreasae in ΔpH^{b-e}.

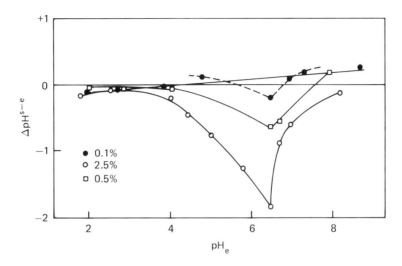

Fig. 1 — The effects of pH_e on ΔpH^{s-e} for Aerosil 200 sols of dispersed phase
concentrations 0.1% (●), 0.5% (□) and 2.5% (○).

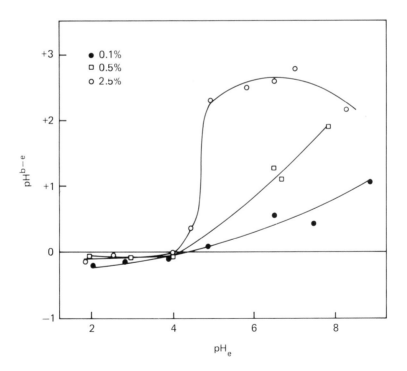

Fig. 2 — The effects of pH_e on ΔpH^{b-e} for Aerosil 200 sols of dispersed phase
concentration 0.1% (●), 0.5% (□) and 2.5% (○).

DISCUSSION

It is clear that quite substantial differences in pH occur between the original pH solutions, the corresponding sols and supernatant liquids. These are noticeable even at the relatively low solid concentrations examined in this work. The two effects of ion-adsorption and the suspension effect can thus produce sizeable errors in pH measurement in these systems.

ΔpH^{s-e} is caused by the suspension effect, whereby there is a difference in pH between the sol itself (which contains charged particles) and its supernatant liquid (which does not contain charged particles). This cannot be interpreted in terms of differing hydrogen ion activities in the two systems [1]. It is due rather to the existence of a higher liquid junction potential when the electrode is immersed in the sol than when it is immersed in the supernatant. The theoretical description of the suspension effect [2] requires that ΔpH^{s-e} be negative in value for negatively-charged dispersed particles. This is indeed the case (Fig. 1).

Any increase in the total amount of surface charge in the system should lead, also on theoretical grounds, to greater values of ΔpH^{s-e}. Thus, larger ΔpH^{s-e} values are observed with increasing solid concentration and hence increasing solid surface area in the sol. Similarly, increase in pH_e above about 3 leads to greater ΔpH^{s-e} values as a result of increasing surface potential [3]. The subsequent decrease in ΔpH^{s-e} above pH_e of 6.5 occurs despite a continued, sharp increase in surface potential in this pH range. This may be due to the increasing ionic strengths of the NaOH solutions used.

With the ΔpH^{b-e} values, the pH of the sol is not included in the calculation. Thus there are no effects due to charged particles, and ΔpH^{b-e} is a measure of the change in hydrogen ion activity caused by the addition of the solid phase. Since these values are positive at pH_e above 3.5, a decrease in pH occurred. This is greater as the solid concentration increases. This is almost certainly owing to loss of hydroxyl ions from the continuum by adsorption on to the solid surface. This occurs in increasing amounts as the pH increases [4].

These experiments confirm that pH_e is the most reliable measure of the hydrogen ion activity of the continuum of suspensions. This is of particular importance, since it is just the pH which influences the zeta potential of charged particles. One must remember that the electrostatic properties of the solid surface are influenced by the pH of the adjacent continuum with which it is in equilibrium. Measurement of the pH of the suspension itself can give pH errors of up to 2 pH units when only 2.5% solid is present in these Aerosil 200 systems. Although this will obviously depend on the nature of the solid phase, pharmaceutical suspensions often contain much higher solid concentrations than those examined here, and substantial errors in pH can therefore occur. Measurement of the pH of the continuum before addition of the solid phase can give errors of a similar magnitude in the systems examined here. This, however, may depend on the nature of any buffers used.

It is thus evident that care should be exercised when measuring the pH of suspensions during their industrial development. The pH is best measured after removal of the dispersed phase by centrifugation. One should be aware of possible errors due to ion adsorption and suspension effects.

REFERENCES

[1] J. Th. G. Overbeek, *J. Coll. Sci.*, **8**, 593 (1953).
[2] Y. M. Chernoberezhskii, *Surface Colloid Sci.*, **11**, 359 (1982).
[3] D. Kerner and W. Leiner, *Coll. Poly. Sci.*, **253**, 960 (1975).
[4] G. H. Bolt, *J. Phys. Chem.*, **61**, 1166 (1957).

12

Control of crystal growth in drug suspensions: design of a control unit and application to acetaminophen suspensions

K. H. Ziller and **H. Rupprecht**
Department of Pharmaceutical Technology, University of Regensburg,
Universitätsstr. 31, D-8400 Regensburg, West Germany

SUMMARY

A control system is described for the monitoring of particle growth by crystallization in pharmaceutical suspensions. The technique is based on the measurement of drug concentration in the liquid phase in contact with the drug crystals. The control unit consists of a thermostated vessel containing the drug suspension and a monitoring circuit including a detector. The concentration of the liquid supernatant is recorded at the same time as the actual temperature. Typical concentration–time curves indicate any dissolution or crystallization if temperature cycling ($\Delta T \pm 10$ K) is applied to the suspensions.

It is shown with acetaminophen crystals that after decreasing the temperature, the crystal growth appears significantly impeded even by very small amounts of polyvinylpyrolidone (PVP) (3 p.p.m., mol mass 180 000). The polymer did not influence the rate of dissolution of the crystals at higher temperatures.

Surfactants reduce the protective action of PVP on crystal growth, in particular anionic surfactants which totally neutralize the protective action.

Crystal growth can be successfully inhibited by substances which are irreversibly adsorbed on to the crystal surface by specific interactions with their functional groups usually using a polymer structure of high molecular mass.

INTRODUCTION

Particle growth by crystallization is one of the most destabilizing physical processes in drug suspensions. It is promoted by temperature changes during storage, especially if the solubility of the drug is strongly dependent on temperature. In this case the crystallized drug may dissolve with increasing temperature, followed by particle growth when the temperature decreases again. Supersaturated drug solutions are then formed, which stimulate crystallization. Crystal growth, however, favours rapid sedimentation and may finally lead to non-redispersible sediments or caking [1].

Several approaches are described in the literature both to monitor these processes and to impede crystallization from supersaturated solutions by the addition of polymers, surfactants, and dyes [2–7]. A control unit is reported in this work which is designed to monitor crystal growth (and dissolution) even in highly-concentrated suspensions. The influence of additives on crystallization processes can also be evaluated.

CONTROL OF SUSPENSION STABILITY

Measurement of particle size

In a suspension the total volume of the solid phase is the sum of the individual volumes of the single particles (i.e. crystals).

Any dissolution or crystallization process will change this solid phase volume. On cooling a drug suspension, particle growth from supersaturated solution may be the preferred process, with the suspended crystals acting as nuclei. Consequently the particle size of the crystals increases. This can be evaluated from measurements of the particle size distribution in the suspension [2,8–10]. Different techniques have been described, for example, the Andreasen pipette [9], the Coulter counter [2,8,10] or the semi- or full automatic particle size determination from microscopic images [4]. However, the analysis of representative samples from pharmaceutical (concentrated) suspensions is more or less an arbitrary procedure. Any pretreatment of the suspensions such as shaking, redispersion etc., as well as the sampling location in the suspension, may alter the particle size values obtained.

An alternative approach is to study crystal growth on single crystals mounted under the microscope. Although this method is very elegant, it may be restricted to fundamental aspects such as the individual growth of different crystal faces, changes in crystal habit, etc. It does not account for the mutual influence of solid particles in real suspensions. In addition, experimental difficulties arise with the need for proper mounting of the crystals and from the necessity to provide a constant and equal flow of the saturated solution around the crystal [4,11,12].

Control of solute concentration in the liquid phase

Sekikawa *et al.* [13] proposed control of crystallization in suspensions by monitoring the concentration of the drug in the liquid phase. In a closed suspension system dissolution and crystallization must change the concentration of the solute in the liquid phase. In this way coprecipitation and particle growth from ethanolic acetaminophen solutions have been controlled by intermittent measurement of the drug concentration in the supernatant liquid. This technique can, however, be improved by continuously controlling the drug concentration in the liquid phase of a suspension both under isothermal and termperature cycling conditions, thereby simulating the stress on storage at varying temperatures.

According to Varney [14] the rate of crystal growth is dependent on a variety of parameters, such as the solubility of the drug (i.e. the saturation concentration) and their temperature dependence, the degree of supersaturation, the temperature difference on storage and the frequency of temperature cycling. Any mechanical stress such as stirring must also be considered. Particles smaller than 1 μm may additionally exhibit Ostwald ripening.

Description of the suspension control unit

The control unit was designed to measure drug concentration in the liquid phase and, simultaneously, the temperature in the suspension. Depending on the monitoring system the concentration of additives influencing the crystallization can also be determined.

The main elements and their function are shown in Fig. 1. A graduated

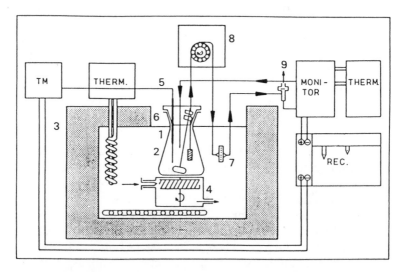

Fig. 1 — System for monitoring the drug concentration in the liquid phase of suspensions during temperature cycling. (1) Stirrer vessel; (2) stirrer with bearing, axis, magnetic pin; (3) heat exchanger (heating and cooling); (4) turbine for the magnetic stirrer drive; (5) temperature sensor; (6) frit; (7) membrane filter; (8) peristaltic pump; (9) septum for sample injection and sampling and bubble removement; TM, temperature control; Therm., thermostat for temperature control of the suspension; Rec., twin-channel recorder.

Erlenmeyer flask with a ground glass stopper (containing connecting tubing) is used as a stirred vessel (1). This contains 50–100 ml of the liquid phase to which the solid drug is added. The suspension is then stirred by a magnetic stirrer (2) at about 300 r.p.m. driven by a magnetic water turbine (4) (Feddeler, Essen, West Germany). Sliding bearings can adjust the stirrer shank in the stopper. The Erlenmeyer flask is contained in a thermostat (temperature adjustment better than ± 0.1 K) and is equipped with heat exchangers for heating and cooling (3) (supplied by a Braun Frigomix 1496/ Thermomix 1480 BKV unit = [Therm]). A Pt-100 sensor (5) connected to a Knauer control unit (TM) controls the temperature in the suspension.

A circuit is then established to control drug (and/or additive) concentrations. The liquid phase is transported through Teflon and Isoversinic tubes by means of a peristaltic pump (Gilson Miniplus (8)). The circuit starts with a glass frit G3 or G4 (6) to trap course solid particles. The liquid then passes through a membrane filter (d_{pore} 8 μm, cellulose nitrate, Sartorius) (7) and a HPLC-septum injector (Perkin–Elmer) (9), so as to remove fine particles and bubbles before passing through the monitor. The monitors used were selected form HPLC equipment. A differential refractometer (Knauer), single beam UV spectrophotometer (Gilson spectrochrome U, Shimadzu UV 102 and UV 100–02), and double beam spectrophotometer (UV 210A Shimadzu) were used.

The flow through cells in the monitor were maintained at temperatures 10 K higher than the upper limiting temperature of any cycle (thermostats). In this way crystallization in the cuvettes is avoided. For UV measurements quartz cells (1–10 mm) were used (Hellma).

The following parameters have to be considered when selecting an appropriate monitor: linearly between the signal and the drug concentration (controlled by calibration), the sensitivity, the signal-to-noise ratio and the thermic drift. Due to the high concentrations in saturated drug solutions, it is better to measure concentration at a wavelength different from the absorption maximum. In this case the validity of the Beer–Lamburt law has to be carefully evaluated. Temperature and concentration signals are recorded in parallel versus time, as is shown in Fig. 2.

The following criteria are necessary for an adequate control of a suspension system:

(a) dissolution and crystallization can be directly controlled by drug concentration without the need for dilution steps;
(b) the rates of dissolution and crystallization are relatively high;
(c) polymorphism and pseudo-polymorphism are excluded;
(d) interaction between drug crystals and excipients are well defined or can be independently determined;
(e) influences on crystal growth can be independently measured by other methods (4–7, 11–13).

Temperature cycling

For one experiment 1–4 g of drug (particle size 10–50 μm) are necessary (suspended in 50–100 ml liquid phase). The experiments are carried out at room temperature — $\Delta T \pm 10$ K — according to the temperature conditions during distribution and storage of the drug preparation. Sixty minutes

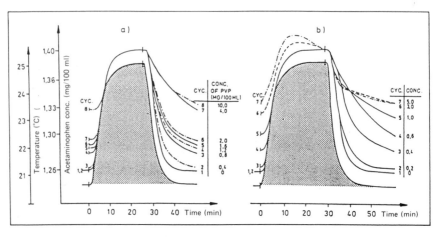

Fig. 2 — Temperature cycling in aqueous acetaminophen suspensions (100 ml, 3%).
(a) Additive PVP K17 (0.4–10 mg/100 ml). (b) Additive PVP K30 (0.2–5 mg/100 ml).
Temperature: curve over the hatched area (also in the following figures).

proved to be a reasonable compromise for one temperature cycle. Considering heating and cooling rates, the length of this temperature plateau phases at the upper limiting temperature (to attain equilibrium) and a cooling period was limited to 30 min.

The control of crystal growth of acetaminophen in the presence of polyvinylpyrolidone

The function and sensitivity of the control unit was evaluated by means of model suspensions in order to evaluate and predict suspension stability. Acetaminophen was selected as a drug model and polyvinylpyrrolidone (PVP) as an effective additive to inhibit crystal growth [4,12,15].

In Fig. 2(a) and (b) dissolution and crystallization of acetaminophen in aqueous suspensions during temperature cycling are demonstrated. PVPs of different molecular mass were added to the suspensions. In the diagrams the temperature and the concentration of the drug in the liquid phase versus the time are given. Locating marks indicate the points of temperature reversal. The number of temperature cycles are listed in the column 'cyc' and the and the concentration of the added PVP in the column 'conc'. During the cooling periods the rate of crystallization obviously decreases with increasing amounts of PVP in the suspensions. Significant influences both on dissolution and crystallization are exhibited by PVP K30 (mol mass $\approx 43\,000$) and PVP K90 (mol mass $\approx 180\,000$) (Fig. 3(a)). The PVP K17 with its lower molecular mass of ≈ 9000, has only a minor influence on these processes.

The number of temperature cycles also influences the effectiveness of PVP. Starting with the fourth cycle, supersaturated solutions are obtained during the dissolution period (related to the solubility at the upper limiting temperature). The concentration passes through a maximum after 8–10 min,

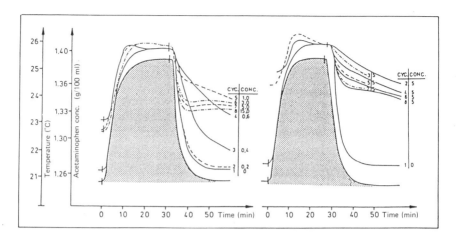

Fig. 3 — Temperature cycling in aqueous acetaminophen suspensions (100 ml, 3%).
(a) Additive PVP K90 (0.2–15 mg/100 ml). (b) Singular addition of 5 mg PVP K90.

then declines to the saturation concentration. Simultaneously the inhibiting action on crystallization) at the lower limiting temperatures) appears more pronounced, and supersaturated suspensions are stabilized over several hours. This is also demonstrated by temperature cycling at constant concentrations of PVP after the second cycle (5 mg/100 ml PVP K90) (Fig. 3(b)). Only a small decrease in concentration is observed during repeated cooling periods.

In Fig. 4 acetaminophen concentrations are shown, obtained during the cooling period of temperature cycling after 10 and 25 min, respectively. They are contrasted with the increasing amounts of PVP K17 and PVP K90 (semilogarithmic plot) added to the system. An effective inhibition of crystallization is indicated by high drug concentrations in the supernatant at low PVP concentrations and by a small difference between the concentration curves at 100 min and 25 min. It is thus confirmed that PVP K90 is a potent crystallization inhibitor. With increasing frequency of temperature cycling the inhibiting action of PVP K90 is reduced to a fairly constant level, even after a further increase of polymer concentration (identical values were obtained by PVP K30, not shown in this diagram). From these experiments it is concluded that approximately 3 mg PVP (= 30 p.p.m.) K30 or K90 is the most effective amount of polymer to inhibit the crystallization of acetaminophen in suspensions.

4-Nitroacetanilide was introduced for comparison as a drug model. The structure of this molecule differs in a *para*-position to the acetamino groups (i.e. the OH group is replaced by a nitro group). In this way the influence of single functional groups on drug crystallization in the presence of PVP can be evaluated (Fig. 5). The inhibitory effect of PVP K30 on the crystallization of 4-nitroacetanilide appears to be smaller, compared with acetaminophen.

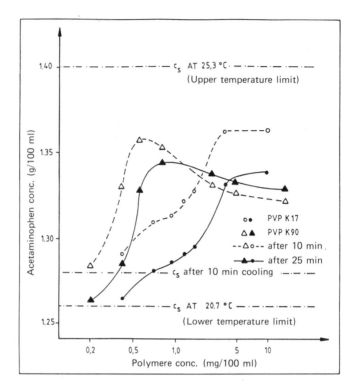

Fig. 4 — Temperature cycling in aqueous acetaminophen suspensions. Drug concentration in the supernatant liquid phase in the presence of: ○--○, PVP K17, 10 min; ○——○, PVP K17, 25 min; △---△, PVP K90, 10 min; △——△, PVP K90, 25 min.

However, bovine serum albumin, a polymer of the protein type is also effective in crystal growth inhibition of 4-nitroacetanilide at concentration of 20 mg/100 ml (=200 p.p.m.). This may be due to the inability of the nitro group to form hydrogen bonds as a donor, leading to weaker interactions with PVP.

Influence of low molecular pyrrolidones, bovine serum albumin and surfactants on acetaminophen crystallization
Addition of 1-methylpyrrolidone and piracetam
The crystallization of acetaminophen during the cooling period in temperature cycling is not significantly influenced by either 1-methylpyrrolidone or piracetam (Fig. 6). Both substances are compounds of similar structure as the pyrrolidone monomers. Even relatively high concentrations of these additives (compared with PVP) are ineffective. During the third cycle PVP K30 was added, and was fully effective even in the presence of both additives. These experiments confirm the results obtained by Mehta [11]. He reported that vinylpyrrolidone does not influence the crystallization of

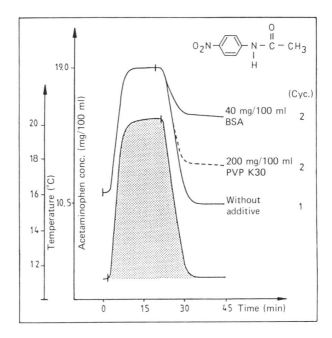

Fig. 5 — Temperature cycling in aqueous 4-nitroacetanilide-suspensions (100 ml, 3%). Additives PVP K30 and BSA.

sulphathiazole, which is also a low molecular mass compound of similar structure. A specific influence of the pyrrolidone ring system on the protective action of PVP can, therefore, be ruled out.

Addition of bovine serum albumin

Bovine serum albumin (BSA) was selected as an example of a polymer which shows strong interactions with a great number of drugs in aqueous solution [15–19]. In Fig. 7 the influence of BSA on acetaminophen concentration in the liquid bulk phase during temperature cycling of the suspension is given. This polymer inhibits the crystallization of acetaminophen to the same extent as PVP.

Combinations of PVP and surfactants

Surfactants are reported to influence crystallization by adsorption and solubilization effects [2,9,10,21,22]. They are also widely used in suspension formulations as wetting agents and preservatives [23]. We studied their possible interference with both the inhibiting polymer [24] and the crystal surfaces during temperature cycling experiments with acetaminophen suspensions. The crystallization of acetaminophen is not influenced by the ionic polyoxyethylene-polypropylene copolymer Pluronic F68.

In combination with PVP K17 the rate of crystallization is only slightly increased by the presence of the surfactant (Fig. 8).

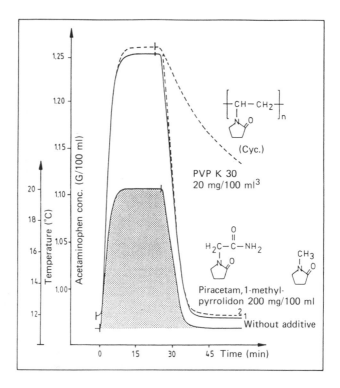

Fig. 6 — Temperature cycling in aqueous acetaminophen suspensions (50 ml, 3%).
Piracetam and 1-methylpyrrolidone, respectively added in the second cycle.

The non-ionic PEG-10-oleylether and hexadecylpyridinium cations both reduce the inhibiting effect of PVP on crystallization (Fig. 9(a) and (b)). These surfactants are reported to exhibit no significant interactions with PVP in solution [25,26], although they may be adsorbed on to the crystal surfaces of the drug. In this way they can disturb the structure of the protective polymer at the crystal surface. Hexadecylsulfate, however, neutralizes the protective action of PVP on acetaminophen crystallization almost completely (Fig. 9(b)). This anionic surfactant aggregates with PVP in the aqueous phase [27], thus preventing the PVP from establishing protective layers on the drug crystals.

DISCUSSION

Specific and storage interactions between functional groups of the drug and a polymer are obviously a necessary, but not a sufficient, prerequisite for the inhibition of crystallization from supersaturated solutions in drug suspensions. This is demonstrated by the low molecular pyrrolidone compounds, which are more or less ineffective in influencing crytallization. The second,

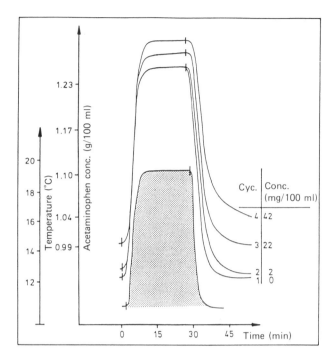

Fig. 7 — Temperature cycling in aqueous acetaminophen suspensions in the presence of BSA (50 ml, 3%).

essential property of a protective substance seems to be the formation of a polymer adsorbate on the surface of the drug crystals. This impedes the approach of drug molecules from solution on to free spaces of the crystal lattice.

In the series of pyrrolidone compounds applied to acetaminophen suspensions, only the high molecular mass polymers (PVP K30, PVP K90) show a pronounced protective action. The adsorption of PVP K17 on acetaminophen crystals is shown in Fig. 10. The Langmuirian nature of the isotherm indicates that the adsorption is reversible, in contrast to the high molecular mass polymers. It can be imagined that the structures of PVP (and BSA) adsorbates formed on acetaminophen from the 'good' solvent, water [28] are responsible for the crystallization-inhibiting effect. The polymer is hydrated to a great extent in the adsorbate and attached to the crystal surface by some segments — so called trains (Fig. 11). Water molecules remain, therefore, in permanent contact with the crystal surface. In raising the temperature the dissolution process can start immediately and drug molecules dissolved from the crystal can diffuse through the adsorbate into the bulk liquid phase.

The inhibiting action of PVP on crystallization is presumably a kinetic effect. PVP inhibits the introduction of drug molecules from solution on to

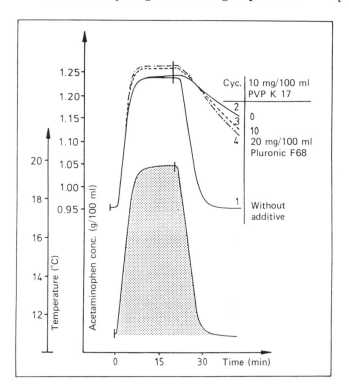

Fig. 8 — Temperature cycling in aqueous acetaminophen suspension (50 ml, 3%) in the presence of PVP K17 and pluronic F68.

the crystal lattice by occupying the adsorption sites which are also free lattice sites. The adsorption of polymers on to solids is known to become progressively more irreversible with increasing chain length [28]. This is also the case if only weak or medium adsorption forces are present on a single adsorption site. For the desorption of a polymer molecule the activation energy of desorption must be simultaneously achieved for every single contact point. In acetaminophen suspension only a gradual replacement of polymer contact sites on the crystals by drug molecules is envisaged. The adsorbed polymer may form a mechanical barrier against crystallization which has increasing protective action by increasing the polymer chain length and, consequently, the irreverisble nature of adsorption.

When applying this method to suspensions of drugs which for polymorphs or pseudo-polymorphs it must be considered that the more stable crystal form may be formed as well as different crystal habits. This could influence the results of the temperature cycling experiments.

The method presented in this chapter may be a useful tool to detect and characterize the influence of additives on drug crystallization in suspensions. Even very small amounts — in the p.p.m. range — show their protective action. It may successfully be applied in the optimization of suspension stability and in the control of these dosage forms.

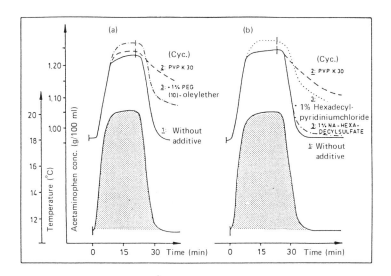

Fig. 9 — Temperature cycling in aqueous acetaminophen suspensions (50 ml, 3%) in the presence of mixtures of PVP K30 (20 mg/100 ml) with (a) PEG(10)oleylether and (b) hexadecylpyridinium chloride and sodium hexadecylsulfate, respectively.

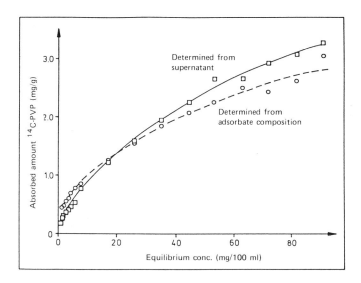

Fig. 10 — Adsorption of PVP (14C-K19/K17 1:50) on to acetaminophen crystals.

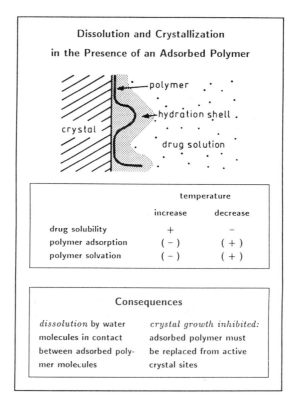

Fig. 11 — Schematic sketch of the polymer adsorbate on a drug crystal and the influence of temperature cycling on the adsorbate.

REFERENCES

[1] A. T. Florence and D. Attwood, in *Physicochemical Principles of Pharmacy*, Macmillan, Houndmills, Basingstoke, London, 1981.

[2] J. E. Carless and A. A. Forster, *J. Pharm. Pharmacol.*, **18**, 697–708 (1966).

[3] M. A. Moustafa, A. R. Ebian, S. A. Khalil and M. M. Motawi, *J. Pharm. Sci.*, **64**, 1485–1489 (1975).

[4] A. P. Simonelli, S. C. Mehta and W. I. Higuchi, *J. Pharm. Sci.*, **59** 633–637 (1970).

[5] B. S. Nath and R. V. Gaitonde, *Ind. J. Pharm.*, **37**, 77–80 (1975).

[6] A. A. Badawi, A. A. El-Sayed and I. Haroun, *Pharm. International*, **5/6**, 1–6 (1977).

[7] E. Nuernberg and P. Kohl, *Pharmaz. Ztg*, **124**, 523–529 (1979).

[8] J. E. Carless, M. A. Moustafa and H. D. C. Rapson, *J. Pharm. Pharmacol.*, **20**, 630–638, 639–645 (1968).

[9] J. Hasegawa and T. Nagai, *Chem. Pharm. Bull.*, **6**, 129–137 (1958).

[10] W. I. Higuchi and P. K. Lau, *J. Pharm. Sci.*, **51**, 1081–1084 (1962).

[11] S. C. Mehta, P. D. Bernardo, W. I. Higuchi and A. P. Simonelli, *J. Pharm. Sci.*, **59**, 638–644 (1970).

[12] S. C. Metha, Ph.D. Thesis Univ. Michigan, 1969.

[13] H. Sekikawa, M. Nakano and T. Arita, *Chem. Pharm. Bull.*, **26**, 118–126 (1978).

[14] G. Varney, *J. Pharm. Pharmacol.*, **19**, (Suppl. 1967). 19s–23s.

[15] A. M. Motawi, S. A. Morbuda, F. El Khawas and K. L. El Khodery, *Acta Pharm. Technol.*, **28**, 211–215 (1982).

[16] C. Davison and P. K. Smith, *J. Pharmacol. Exptl. Therap.*, **133** 161–170 (1961).

[17] M. L. Eichman, D. E. Guttman, Q. van Winkle and E. P. Guth, *J. Pharm. Sci.*, **51**, 66–71 (1962).

[18] P. M. Keen, *Brit. J. Pharmacol.*, **26** 704–712 (1966).

[19] A. Lindenbaum and J. Schubert, *J. Phys. Chem.*, **60**, 1663–1665 (1956).

[20] N. K. Patel, P.-C. Sheen and K. E. Taylor, *J. Pharm. Sci.*, **57**, 1370–1374 (1968).

[21] A. S. Michaels and A. R. Colville, *J. Phys. Chem.*, **64**, 13–19 (1960).

[22] A. S. Michaels and F. W. Tausch, *J. Phys. Chem.*, **65**, 1730–1734 (1961).

[23] W. I. Higuchi, J. Swarbrick, F. H. Norman, A. P. Simonelli and A. Martin, 'Particle phenomena and coarse dispersions', in *Remington's Pharmaceutical Sciences* 17th edn.; A. R. Geunaro, Mack Publishing Comp., Easton Pa, 1985, pp. 301.

[24] S. Saito, 'Polymer surfactant interactions', in *Nonionic Surfactants*, M. J. Schick (ed.), Marcel Dekker, New York, Basel, 1987, pp. 881.

[25] S. Saito, *Koll.-Z. u. Z. Polymere*, **249**, 1096–1100 (1971).

[26] S. Saito and K. Kitamura, *J. Coll. Int. Sci.*, **35**, 346–353 (1971).

[27] S. Saito, T. Taniguchi and K. Kitamura, *J. Coll. Int. Sci.*, **37** 154–164 (1971).

[28] T. F. Tadros in *Polymer Coolloids*, R. Buscall, T. Corner and J. F. Stageman (eds), Elsevier Applied Sci. Publ., London, New York, 1985, pp. 105.

13

Water vapour interaction with pharmaceutical cellulose powders

G. R. Sadeghnejad, P. York and **N. G. Stanley-Wood***
Postgraduate Schools of Pharmacy and *Powder Technology University of Bradford, Bradford, West Yorkshire BD7 1DP, UK

SUMMARY

Since interaction between water and particulate solid is a major factor in formulation, processing and product performance of pharmaceuticals, the moisture sorption properties of four grades of microfine cellulose (MFC) and three grades of microcrystalline cellulose (MCC) were investigated. All the powders investigated exhibited type II BDDT sorption isotherms, from which the monolayer capacity and surface area could be evaluated. The heat of sorption ($-\Delta H_a$) and immersion ($-\Delta H_i$) of water vapour were determined by batch and flow microcalorimetry, which together with the water sorption isotherms gave the integral ($-\Delta H$) and differential heats ($-\overline{\Delta H}$), free energies ($-\overline{\Delta F}$) and entropies ($-\overline{\Delta S}$) of sorption. This investigation showed that $-\overline{\Delta H}$ of MFC P050 with a nitrogen surface area of 1.85 mg^{-1} and MCC PH 101 with a nitrogen surface area of 1.22 m^2 g^{-1} were -39.5 and -37.08 kJ mole^{-1} of water respectively.

The generally used Braunauer, Emmett and Teller (BET) relationship in describing full water sorption isotherms was found to be unsatisfactory, but the Guggenheim, Anderson and de Boer (GAB) equation was discriminative and meaningful and could be used to give the thermodynamic energetic constants, C_G and K from the various celluloses.

INTRODUCTION

Cellulose powders are widely used in the pharmaceutical industry as excipients, disintegrants, binders for encapsulation and anti-adherents. The interaction of water with pharmaceutical excipients is important in the ultimate release of drugs and the storage conditions of dosage forms.

A review of the literature on pharmaceutical cellulose powders revealed differences in external surface areas when measured by different adsorbents such as nitrogen and water vapour. Hollenbeck *et al.* [1] determined the surface area of microcrystalline cellulose (MCC) (Avicel PH 101) by the adsorption method for nitrogen and water vapour. Surface areas calculated from the BET equation from adsoprtion isotherms of 1 $m^2 g^{-1}$ and 130 $m^2 g^{-1}$ were found by nitrogen and water sorption respectively. Nakai *et al.* [2] similarly measured the surface area of MCC PH 101 by nitrogen and water sorption and obtained figures of 1 $m^2 g^{-1}$ and 149 $m^2 g^{-1}$ respectively. Van den Berg [3], describing in more detail water sorption on dry starch, emphasized the importance of the state of equilibrium. He suggested that this analysis led to a model of sorption which could serve as a basis for further analysis using existing theories and developed hypotheses. Zografi *et al.* [4] suggested that the BET equation should be extended and applied, and by using polymer solution theory, water sorption should be treated as a hydration process.

As shown in the work of Van den Berg [3] with starch, the BET relationship has been extended according to an equation developed by Anderson [5] and Guggenheim [6] and de Boer [7], referred to as the GAB equation (equation 1); Here W is the weight of water absorbed, C_G and K are constants, W_m is the weight of water forming monolayer and p/p_0 is the relative humidity.

$$W = \frac{C_G . K . W_m p/p_0}{(1 - Kp/p_0)(1 - Kp/p_0 + C_G Kp/p_0)} \qquad (1)$$

The GAB equation was derived to take into account layers of sorbed vapour having properties intermediate to those in the first layer and those of bulk water. The GAB equation is similar to the BET equation, except for the addition of a third parameter, K, that can be determined by equation (2).

$$K = B \exp \frac{H_L - H_m}{RT} \qquad (2)$$

where B is constant, H_L is the heat of liquefaction, and H_m is the heat of sorption of water sorbed in the intermediate layer. The constant C_G can be determined as

$$C_G = D \exp \frac{H_1 - H_m}{RT} \qquad (3)$$

where D is a constant, H_1 is the heat of sorption of water in the first sorbed layer and H_m is the heat of sorption of water sorbed in the intermediate layer. The general character of the GAB analysis has also been realized recently by Dent [8] and Gascoyne and Pethig [9], who applied the GAB equation to consider water vapour sorption on biopolymers.

The object of this work was to determine the surface energetics of different sources of cellulose powders and to examine the mechanism of interaction and distribution pattern for sorbed water molecules in these materials.

EXPERIMENTAL

Materials
Two different types of high grade pharmaceutical celluloses were examined (a) microfine cellulose, MFC (Elcema P050, P100, F150 and granulated G250, Degussa), products obtained by a milling process, (b) microcrystalline cellulose, MCC (Avicel PH 105, 102, 101, FMC Corporation) obtained by spray drying.

Methods
Low temperature nitrogen adsorption. The surface areas of MFC and MCC powders were determined by nitrogen adsorption at 77.5 K. The apparatus used was a glass apparatus similar to British Standard specification [10].

Water vapour sorption: The water vapour sorption isotherms and surface area of MFC and MCC powders were determined at 20°C using equipment based on that previously described by Okhamafe and York [11]. All samples were dried at 70°C and evacuated overnight to a vacuum of 1×10^{-4} torr.

Heats of immersion and sorption: The heats of immersion and sorption of MFC and MCC ar 20°C were measured using an LKB microcalorimeter (model 2107). The LKB microcalorimeter was operated in a batch mode to determine the heats of immersion and in a flow mode at various humidities in the range 5–75% RH to determine the heats of sorption using standard procedures.

RESULTS AND DISCUSSION

Figures 1 and 2 represent the water vapour sorption isotherms for MFC and MCC grades respectively. Analysis of the water vapour sorption data as well as nitrogen absorption data for MFC and MCC indicated that the BET theory [12] can be applied in the range of 5–35% RH. Comparison of surface areas for MFC and MCC obtained from nitrogen adsoprtion and water sorption (see Table 1) showed an approximate relationship for $S_{BET}^{H_2O}/S_{BET}^{N_2}$ of 100 for the materials examined. Young and Healy [13] have observed a similar phenomenon with asbestos powders. Hollenbeck *et al.* [1] suggested that the difference between the size of the nitrogen and water molecules is not sufficient to justify the hundred-fold difference observed. However Zografi *et al.* [4] criticized Hollenbeck *et al*'s explanation that frozen water was blocking the access of nitrogen to MCC pores at the temperature of liquid nitrogen. An alternative explanation is to consider that water interacts with the anhydroglucose molecule in the cellulose polymer chain. In this case the surface area obtained by water sorption should not be regarded as a

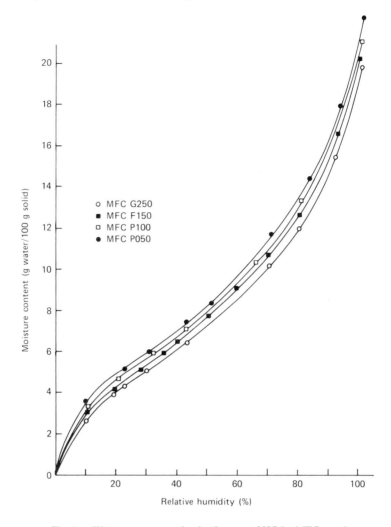

Fig. 1 — Water vapour sorption isotherms at 20°C for MFC powders.

true internal surface, because the surface area evaluated reflects sorption and the phenomenon of water association with the anhydroglucose molecules. In contrast, the nitrogen adsorption technique measures by physical adsoprtion the internal and external surface. As indicated in Table 1, a linear relationship was found for MFC and MCC grades when the weight of water sorbed at various RH was plotted versus nitrogen volume adsorbed at the same relative pressures. The plot also showed the quantity of water sorbed was much greater than for nitrogen and thus the affinity of the physical surface for the water molecules is greater than for the nitrogen molecules. The concept of frozen water present on the surface of the solid in the case of MFC and MCC grades is therefore untenable.

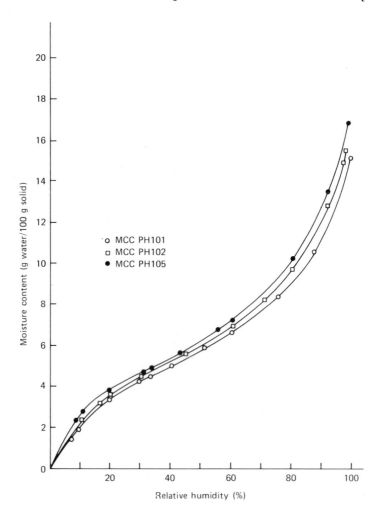

Fig. 2 — Water vapour sorption isotherms at 20°C for MCC powders.

In order to analyse the sorption isotherms over a wider range of RH, the GAB equation was used. Figures 3 and 4 plotting $1/W$ versus p/p_0 demonstrate the fit of experimental data to the GAB equation. Derived constants W_m, C_G and K together with V_m and C constants from the BET equation are listed in Table 2. The data show that the results obtained with the BET and the GAB isotherm equations for values of V_m and C, and W_m and G_G respectively are comparable. However, the monolayer values from the GAB equation are considerably higher.

For a test of physical significance, the heat of liquefaction (H_L), and heat of sorption of water in the intermediate layer (H_m) can be determined from equations (2) and (3) respectively and compared with the value obtained

Table 1 — Surface areas of cellulose powders by nitrogen adsorption and water vapour sorption

Sample	Surface area by N_2 adsorption S_2^N (m^2g^{-1}) BET	Surface area by water vapour sorption S^{H_2O} (m^2g^{-1}) BET
MFC P050	1.85	196
MFC P100	1.58	171
MFC F150	1.39	167
MFC Granulated	0.89	165
MCC PH 105	2.45	173
MCC PH 102	1.12	117
MCC PH 101	1.22	139

calorimetrically [1, 3, 14]. Table 3 shows the values of $H_1 - H_L$ and $H_m - H_L$, assuming B and D to be unity, with calorimetric values presumed to represent sorption in the first and second layers. A reasonable order of magnitude agreement between GAB theoretical and calorimetric experimental values was observed, although not unexpectedly, the $H_m - H_L$ values did exhibit significant differences.

The integral and differential Gibbs' free energy changes associated with the sorption of water vapour on MFC and MCC powders were calculated from the moisture content and values of relative humidities taken at selected intervals from the water sorption isotherms (Figs. 1 and 2) using the relationships reported by Hollenbeck et al. [1]. The integral Gibbs' free energy changes were calculated using equation (4).

$$- \Delta F = n_1 RT \ln p/p_0 - RT\int n_1 \, d(\ln p/p_0) \qquad (4)$$

where n_1 is a number of moles of water sorbed and R is the gas constant, T is temperature, p is the actual vapour pressure and p_0 is the vapour pressure of pure liquid. The integral part of the equation can be obtained graphically by plotting $n_1 \, p_0/p$ and p/p_0 and determining the area under the graph to the upper limiting value of p/p_0 which is required.

$$- RT \int_0^{p/p_0} n_1 d(\ln p/p_0) = - RT \int_0^{p/p_0} \frac{n_1 p_0}{p} \, d(p/p_0) \qquad (5)$$

The differential Gibbs' free energy changes were determined from equation (6).

$$- \overline{\Delta F} = RT \ln p/p_0 \qquad (6)$$

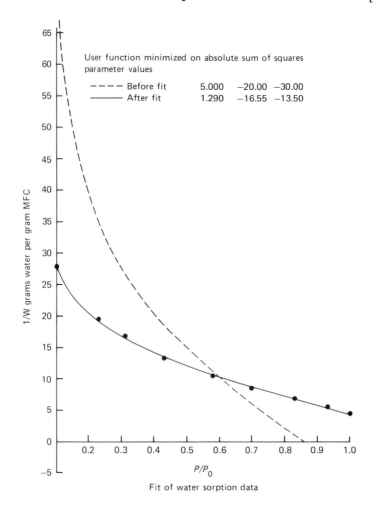

Fig. 3 — Fit of water sorption data for batch A MFC P050 to GAB equation.

The net integral enthalpies ($-\Delta H$) were calculated for both MFC P050 and MCC PH 101 using equation (7).

$$-\Delta H = \Delta H_s - (-n_1\lambda) \tag{7}$$

where H_s is the heat of sorption obtained from flow microcalorimetry. Entropy changes associated with the sorption process were determined by equation (8).

$$\Delta S = \frac{\Delta H - \Delta F}{T} \tag{8}$$

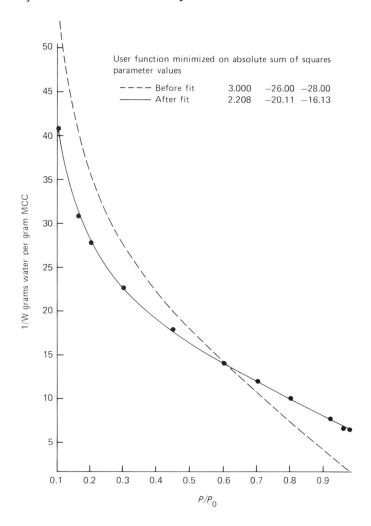

Fig. 4 — Fit of water sorption data for MCC PH 101 to GAB equation.

Figures 5 and 6 illustrate the relationship between the integral thermodynamic functions and the amount of water vapour sorbed for MFC P050 and MCC PH 101 respectively. All curves in Figs. 5 and 6 show an increase asymptotically approaching a limiting value which corresponds to the maximum moisture sorbed. However the values $-\Delta F$, $-\Delta H$ and ΔS in its current form do not differentiate the effect and sorption of each n mole of water vapour has on the change of the thermodynamic state functions. Therefore, the thermodynamic state functions were differentiated with respect to the amount of water vapour sorbed and these values are illustrated in Figs. 7 and 8 for MFC P050 and MCC PH 101. The curves for MCC

Table 2 — BET and GAB equation data for all grades at MFC and MCC powders

Sample	BET equation paratemeters		GAB equation parameters			Number of data points
	V_m	C	W_m	C_G	K	
MFC P050	0.425	12.27	0.0696	18.66	0.770	9
MFC P100	0.363	10.80	0.0520	17.59	0.772	8
MFC F150	0.319	11.12	0.0484	16.99	0.784	11
MFC Granulated G250	0.205	15.10	0.0500	11.62	0.765	10
MCC PH 105	0.563	35.47	0.0423	18.74	0.761	10
MCC PH 102	0.257	42.63	0.0443	10.98	0.710	10
MCC PH 101	0.280	29.29	0.0420	14.28	0.742	11

Table 3 — Comparison of values of enthalpy of sorption obtained from calorimetric experiments and the GAB equation

Sample	GAB (kcal/mole)		Calorimetric (kcal/mole)	
	$H_m - H_L$	$H_1 - H_L$	$H_m - H_L$	$H_1 - H_L$
MFC P050	0.153	1.867	4.2	1.3
MFC P100	0.151	1.830		
MFC F150	0.142	1.800		
MFC Granulated G250	0.157	1.593		
MCC PH 105	0.160	1.875		
MCC PH 102	0.200	1.673		
MCC PH 101	0.174	1.731	3.6	1.2

PH 101 are similar to those reported previously by Hollenbeck et al. [1]. The curves show that:

(1) $-\overline{\Delta H}$ is constant up to values approaching monolayer with respect to anhydroglucose molecules suggesting an energetically homogeneous surface available for water vapour molecules and may represent the extent of an interaction between a single water vapour molecule with each anhydroglucose molecule;

(2) the second region shows a steady fall in $-\overline{\Delta H}$ after a discontinuity between $n_1 = 0.18$ and 0.22, which suggests weaker bonding of water molecules with less homogeneity of the water–anhydroglucose interaction. This region may be associated with a second sorbed water molecule per anhydroglucose residue;

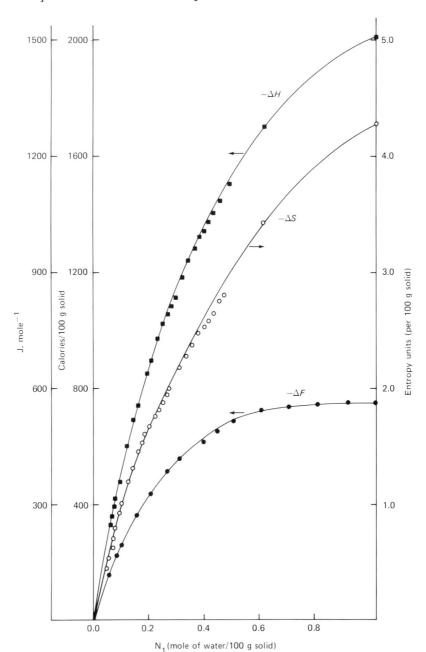

Fig. 5 — Integral thermodynamic properties of sorption at 20°C for MFC P050.

(3) at higher values of n_1 (>0.5), $-\overline{\Delta H}$ falls steadily to low values indicating the uptake of non-specific bulk water.

The differential heat of sorption ($-\overline{\Delta H}$) of water on MCC showed similar

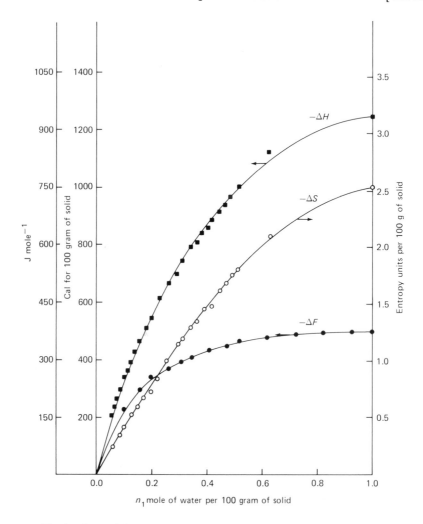

Fig. 6 — Integral thermodynamic properties of sorption for the MCC PH 101.

regions but gave smaller values of $-\overline{\Delta H}$, $-\overline{\Delta F}$ and $-\overline{\Delta S}$ than MFC P050. The different numerical values between these products may reflect the different crystallinity of the two materials, MFC and MCC, with water vapour sorption occurring only in the amorphous cellulose regions. Morrison and Dzieciuch [14] examining moisture sorption on powders, concluded that the initial decrease of $-\overline{\Delta H}$ was due to a peptization (swelling) of the solid. The energy consumed in the disruption of solid–liquid bonds, produced a non-constant and lower heat of sorption than expected. This effect, which is carried implicitly throughout the determination of $-\Delta H$ from immersional data, is not present in the study of MFC and MCC. Therefore, the constant $-\overline{\Delta H}$ period seems to be an indication of zero swelling as well as an indication of an energetically homogeneous surface [1].

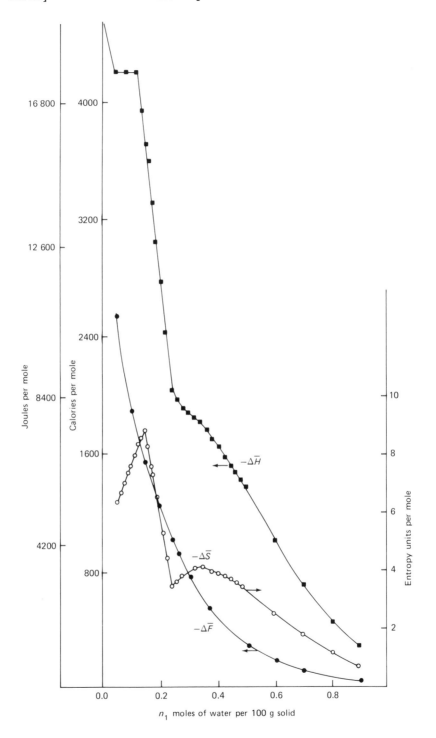

Fig. 7 — Differential thermodynamic properties of MFC P050.

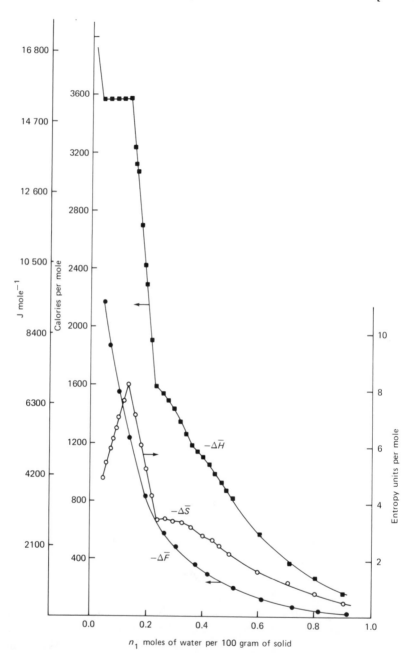

Fig. 8 — Differential thermodynamic properties of MCC PH 101.

The differential entropy at very low moisture content (Figs. 7 and 8) is positive. The increase in the ordered system is greatest when the first water molecule interacts with the anhydroglucose molecule. After that the rate of ordering diminishes but is still positive. As more moisture is sorbed, however, the differential entropy will continually decrease. The continuous increase in the negative differential entropy value is a result of a decrease in the sorption of water molecules in the surface film. The increase in the negative differential entropy corresponds to a period of accelerated ordering, due primarily to the approach of monolayer completion.

To examine the water sorption sequence further the differential heat of sorption obtained microcalorimetially ($\overline{\Delta H_a}$) was correlated with the moisture content of the powders. The graph of $-\overline{\Delta H_a}$ versus moisture content illustrated in Fig. 9 indicates three sections and these can be distinguished

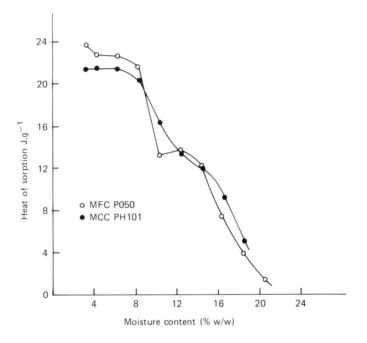

Fig. 9 — Differential heat of sorption versus moisture content for MCC PH 101 and MFC P050.

both for MFC P050 and MCC PH 101. In MCC an initial constant level of $-\overline{\Delta H_a}$ occurs from 3–7% w/w moisture content indicating very strong sorbed water. A second plateau, less defined but still distinguishable, is observed at a lower $-\overline{\Delta H_a}$ between 10–14% w/w. Above this moisture level, the continuous decrease in $-\overline{\Delta H_a}$ suggests that the sorbed water begins to resemble bulk water. The discontinuities in the curve correspond to stoichiometric ratios of approximately 1:1 and 2:1 of water to anhydroglucose unit assuming a crystallinity figure of 63% [15] and that moisture is taken up by the amorphous regions of cellulose [16]. The presence of these plateau regions thus supports the sorption model of a stronger specific interaction of a single water vapour molecule per anhydroglucose molecule followed after completion by a weaker interaction by a second water vapour molecule with each anhydroglucose molecule in the amorphous region. For MFC the values of $-\overline{\Delta H_a}$ over the plateau regions are more clearly defined than for MCC. These differences between cellulose powders can be attributed to differences in powder pretreatment, inducing, for example, different degrees of crystallinity or surface energies.

The observations from this microcalorimetric study thus clearly support the interpretation and hypotheses put forward by the GAB equation and sorption isotherm analysis. It is interesting to note that the model proposed by Van den Berg [3] for water sorption in starch powders, appears to also hold for cellulose powders.

REFERENCES

[1] G. Hollenbeck, G. E. Peck and D. O. Kildsig, *J. Pharm. Sci.*, **67**, 1599 (1978).

[2] Y. Nakai, E. Fukuoka, S. Nakajimi and K. Yamamoto, *Chem. Pharm. Bull.*, **25** (10), 2490 (1977).

[3] C. Van den Berg, Vapour sorption equilibria and other water-starch interactions, physico-chemical approach. Agricultural University of Wageningen, the Netherlands, pp. 26–31, 33, 55–57, 65, 85–91, 94–99 (1981).

[4] G. Zografi, M. J. Kontny, A. Y. S. Yang and G. S. Brenner, *Int. J. Pharm.*, **18**, 99 (1984).

[5] R. B. Anderson, *J. Am. Chem. Soc.*, **68**, 686 (1946).

[6] E. A. Guggenheim (ed.), *Application of Statistical Mechanics*. Clarendon Press, Oxford, pp. 186–206 (1966).

[7] J. H. de Boer (ed.), *The Dynamical Character of Adsorption*, 2nd edn., Clarendon Press, Oxford, pp. 20–219 (1968).

[8] R. W. Dent, *Text. Res.*, **J47**, 145 (1977).

[9] P. R. C. Gascoyne and R. Pethig, *J. Chem. Soc., Faraday Trans.*, 1, **73**, 171 (1977).

[10] British Standard Specification, Part 1, 4359 (1969).

[11] A. O. Okhamafe and P. York, *J. Pharm. Pharmacol.*, **35**, 409 (1983).

[12] S. Brunauer, P. H. Emmett and E. J. Teller, *Am. Chem. Soc.*, **60**, 309 (1938).

[13] G. J. Young and F. H. Healy, *J. Phys. Chem.*, **58**, 881 (1954).

[14] J. L. Morrison and M. A. Dzieciuch, *Can. J. Chem.*, **37**, 1379 (1959).

[15] Y. Nakai, E. Fukuoka, S. Nakajima and J. Hasegawa, *Chem. Pharm. Bull.*, **25**, 96 (1977).

[16] A. J. Stamm, *Wood and Cellulose Science,* Ronald Press, New York (1964).

14

Determination of dielectric properties and adsorption isotherms of water adsorbed on to Fractosil 5000

Vo Van Nhuan, M. Buchmann, C. Rey-Mermet, P. Ruelle, Hô Nam-Trân and U. W. Kesselring
Institute of Pharmaceutical Analysis, School of Pharmacy, University of Lausanne, Place du Château 3, 1005 Lausanne, Switzerland

INTRODUCTION

In a solid state pharmaceutical preparation, the water adsorbed on the surfaces of the drugs and of the excipients generally reduces the stability of the active constituents [1]. It has been established that only part of the total amount of water influences degradation kinetics [2] and that this depends on the physicochemical state of the water. Thus, in order to understand the part played by the water adsorbed, it is of prime importance to know its exact amount in the system and to characterize it quantitatively by measurable parameters. Two experimental methods have been used in the present work to investigate the properties of the water at the surface. First, the adsorption isotherm has been chosen as the appropriate method to obtain the information related to the thermodynamic properties of water. For this purpose, frontal chromatography [3] has been used. Not only does it yield results as precise as those obtained by thermogravimetry, but, moreover, it is a much faster method. Furthermore, when an excipient substantially adsorbs water vapour, frontal chromatography is superior to elution adsorption chromatography, since it permits the attainment of better thermodynamic equilibrium in the column.

Secondly, the water/excipient system was also considered as a macroscopic entity of which the dielectric properties were investigated to determine the relaxation parameters of the movement of the water molecules at the surface. Those parameters include the relaxation time, the relaxation activation enthalpy and entropy considered as a function of the amount of water adsorbed on the solid.

The aim of the present work was to describe and evaluate the construction of two sample conditioning devices:

(a) A saturation system coupled to a chromatograph to obtain the water adsorption isotherms on Fractosil® 5000 silica; a good model substance with well determined porosity and granulometry (mean porous diameter: 5000 Å, partial size distribution: 0.063–0.125 mm).

(b) An experimental set-up including a capacitance cell filled with Fractosil® 5000 for the dielectric measurements over a wide frequency range: 100 Hz to 13 MHz.

Various parameters can be derived from the water adsorption isotherms and these include:

— the amount of water adsorbed by 1 g of adsorbent, r (g/g), as a function of the relative humidity, p/p_0, and of the temperature, $T(K)$.

— the specific surface, Σ_{H_2O}, as well as the net monolayer enthalpy, ΔH_{net};

— the variation of some thermodynamic quantities (isosteric enthalpy, isosteric entropy, free energy) as a function of the degree of coverage expressed in number of layers, θ;

— the relative quantity of free- (condensation) and bound water (solvation). The data were analysed according to the BET method [4] and the Hailwood–Horrobin model [5]. The isosteric enthalpy and entropy were calculated according to King and Woodruff [6]. As for the dielectric data, they were dealt with according to the Debye relaxation model [7] and represented by the Cole–Cole [8] diagram, according to Eyring's [9] model.

The dielectric method reveals the existence of three distinct states of water adsorbed onto Fractosil 5000.

THEORETICAL

Adsorption isotherms by frontal chromatography [3]

The principle of frontal chromatography [3] consists of letting a non-adsorbed carrier gas (helium) circulate through the sample until the baseline is stable. Then, at time t_0, the carrier gas is replaced by a water/carrier gas mixture at the same flow rate, D_s, and a C_s concentration in water. Adsorption equilibrium is reached once the height of the platform of the chromatogram no longer varies with time. At time t_1, the gas/water flow is replaced by pure carrier gas. This change is recorded on the chromatogram as the beginning of the desorption curve and the return to the base-line shows the end of the desorption.

From Fig. 1, the hatched area, A_{ads}, is proportional to the quantity of water adsorbed by the sample, whereas the dotted area, A_{des}, is pro-

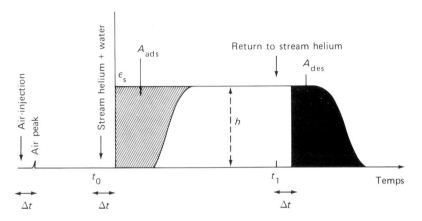

Fig. 1 — Frontal chromatographic diagram.

portional to the quantity of water released from the sample during desorption. If the phenomenon is reversible

$$A_{ads} = A_{des} \qquad (1)$$

The quantity, r, of water adsorbed on the sample is calculated from the chromatographic conditions imposed [3,10] as well as from the characteristics of the chromatogram

$$r = (MD_s/mVRh')(1/T_a)(P_a/P_c)pA_{ads} \qquad (2)$$

where r is the relative quantity of water adsorbed on the adsorbent (g/g), M is the molar mass of water (18 g/mol), D_s is the flow rate of carrier gas (ml/min), m is the mass of adsorbent in the column (g), R is the perfect gas constant (82.057 cm³ atm K⁻¹), V is the chart paper rate (cm/min), h' is the height of chromatographic platform (cm), P_a is the ambient pressure (atm), T_a is the room temperature (K), P_c is the pressure within the column (atm), p is the partial pressure of water according to temperature tables [14] (atm) and A_{ads} is the adsorption surface (cm²).

The adsorption isotherm at a given temperature is obtained by plotting r versus p/p_0.

Specific surface, Σ_{H_2O} (m²/g)
The specific surface is calculated from results obtained from the BET model.

$$\frac{p/p_0}{r \cdot (1 - p/p_0)} = \frac{1}{C \cdot r_m} + \frac{C-1}{C \cdot r_m} p/p_0 \qquad (3)$$

$$C = e^{(q_1 - q_L)/RT} \qquad (4)$$

$$\Sigma_{H_2O} = r_m/M \cdot A_m N 10^{-20} \tag{5}$$

where

p/p_0 = relative humidity (percentage)
r = quantity of water adsorbed at a given humidity (g/g)
C = BET constant
$q_1 - q_L$ = net adsorption heat (kcal/mol); q_1 = isosteric heat of adsorption;
       q_L = heat of condensation (10.55 kcal/mol)
r_m = quantity of water in the first layer (g/g)
N = Avogadro number (6.02252×10^{23} mol^{-1})
A_m = molecular area of water (10.6 Å^2)
M = molar mass of water (18 g/mol).

The plot of $p/p_0/[r(1 - p/p_0]$ versus p/p_0 should therefore be a straight line with a $(C-1)/r_m C$ slope and a $1/r_m C$ intercept. The solution of these two simultaneous equations yields r_m and C, which are used to calculate Σ_{H_2O} and $q_1 - q_L$.

The Hailwood-Horrobin [5] sorption model

This sorption theory was applied by Hailwood and Horrobin [5], to study the water adsorption on textile fibres such as wool, silk and cotton. The model chosen is based on the supposition that the adsorbed water exists in two states: pure liquid water and water combined with the fibre molecules to form a hydrate. It is then simply assumed that the three species present in the solid phase — dissolved water, unhydrated molecules and hydrated molecules — form an ideal solid solution. Assuming that this solid solution phase is in equilibrium with the water vapour phase, Hailwood–Horrobin derived an isotherm model described by the following equation:

$$H/100r = A + BH - C'H^2 \tag{6}$$

where

    $H = 100\, p/p_0$ (relative humidity in percentage)
    r = quantity of water adsorbed per 1 g of adsorbent (g/g).

The three coefficients A, B and C' are determined by a multilinear regression of $H/100r$ against 1, H and H^2.

The Hailwood–Horrobin model permits separate calculation of the relative quantities of free water, r_1 (condensation), and bound water, r_2 (solvation), the sum of which is equal to the total amount of water, r, adsorbed per 1 g of solid.

$$r_1 = (H/(1 - \alpha H))(1/(1 + \beta)A) \tag{7}$$

$$r_2 = (H/(1 + \alpha\beta H))(\beta/(1 + \beta)A) \tag{8}$$

where

$$\alpha = [-B + (B^2 + 4AC')^{1/2}]/2A$$
$$\beta = C'/A\alpha^2$$

The theory of gas–solid chromatography is based on the existence of an adsorption equilibrium between the tridimensional gas phase and the bidimensional adsorbed phase.

The relevant thermodynamic parameters of adsorbed water may be estimated by the three following equations:

The isosteric enthalpy of adsorption, ΔH_{iso}, is deduced from the equation [6]:

$$(\ln p)_r = \Delta H_{iso}/RT + \text{Const} \tag{9}$$

p being the partial water vapour pressure at a fixed amount of adsorbed water r.

The isosteric entropy of adsorption, ΔS_{iso}, is calculated according to [6]:

$$\Delta S_{iso} = \Delta H_{iso}/T + R \ln (p/p_0) \tag{10}$$

The isosteric free energy of adsorption, ΔG_{iso}, is deduced from the general equation:

$$\Delta G_{iso} = \Delta H_{iso} - T\Delta S_{iso} \tag{11}$$

Dielectric relaxation
The fundamental equation of the modified Debye model [8] linking dielectric constants and relaxation times is:

$$\varepsilon^* = \varepsilon' - i\varepsilon'' = \varepsilon^\infty + \frac{\varepsilon_s - \varepsilon^\infty}{1 + (1\omega\tau_0)^{1-\alpha}} \tag{12}$$

with

$$\varepsilon' = C_d/C_0 \quad \text{and} \quad \varepsilon'' = D_x\varepsilon'$$

ε^* is the complex dielectric constant and ε' and ε'' are its real and imaginary parts, C_d is the capacitance (pf) of the cell filled with the dielectric substance in equilibrium with water vapour at various relative humidities, C_0 is the capacitance (pf) of the empty cell and D_x is the loss tangent ($\varepsilon''/\varepsilon'$), ε_s, ε^∞ are respectively the static and infinite frequency dielectric constants, i the imaginary operator and ω the angular frequency, given by $\omega = 2\pi\nu$, ν being the oscillation frequency (Hz) of the electric field, τ_0 is the most probable relaxation time (s) of the water adsorbed and α is a parameter varying from 0 to 1, which measures the degree of departure from an ideal Debye behaviour ($\alpha = 0$).

Transformations of equation (12) give:

$$\varepsilon'' = -bc' + (b^2 (1 + c'^2) - (\varepsilon' - a)^2)^{1/2} \qquad (13)$$

where

$$a = (\varepsilon_s + \varepsilon_\infty)/2$$
$$b = (\varepsilon_s - \varepsilon_\infty)/2$$
$$c' = \cotg [\pi/2 (1 - \alpha)]$$

Experimental measurements provide the C_0, C_d and D_x values as a function of frequency and a non-linear regression yields the constants a, b and c' and hence ε_s and ε_∞. For the non-linear regression calculation, a BASIC computer program developed according to Marquardt's [15] algorithm was used.

A plot of ε'' versus ε' is called a Cole–Cole [8] diagram (Fig. 2).

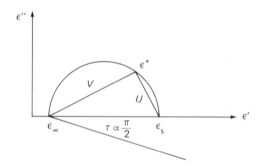

Fig. 2 — Cole–Cole diagram.

The two complex numbers $V = \varepsilon^* - \varepsilon_\infty$ and $U = \varepsilon^* - \varepsilon_s$ are represented by two arc chords plotted on the Cole–Cole diagram.

The relaxation time, τ_0, is calculated from the modification of equation (12):

$$\ln|V/U| = (\alpha - 1) \ln \omega + (\alpha - 1) \ln \tau_0 \qquad (14)$$

The linear regression of $\ln |U/V|$ against $\ln \omega$ yields the two parameters α and τ_0.

If the dipole rotation of a water molecule involves a free energy of activation separating its two mean equilibrium positions, the relaxation activation enthalpy, $\Delta H_\varepsilon^{\neq}$, can be calculated from the temperature dependence of the characteristic frequency, ν_0, defined by $\nu_0 = 1/2\pi\tau_0$ (Eyring's [9] model).

The relaxation activation enthalpy, $\Delta H_\varepsilon^{\neq}$ can be obtained by means of equation (5):

$$\Delta H_\varepsilon^{\neq} = -Rd/(d(1/T)) \log v_0 - RT \tag{15}$$

Once $\Delta H_\varepsilon^{\neq}$ and τ_0 are known, the relaxation activation entropy $\Delta S_\varepsilon^{\neq}$ is given by:

$$\Delta S_\varepsilon^{\neq} = \Delta H_\varepsilon^{\neq}/T + R \ln[(kT\tau_0)/h] \tag{16}$$

The constants R, k, h and T have their usual dimensions and meanings.

EXPERIMENTAL

Instrumental device for frontal chromatography

In frontal chromatography, the chromatograph is coupled to a saturation system. To establish the isotherms, it is necessary adequately to equilibrate the sample substance, used as the stationary phase in the column, with water vapour of precisely known pressure supplied by the saturation system (Fig. 3).

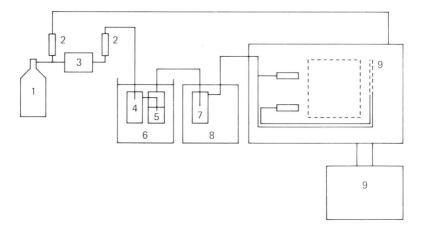

Fig. 3 — Block scheme of the saturation system connected to a gas-chromatograph. (1) Pure helium source (He 99.996), (2) flow rate regulator, (3) pressure regulator, (4) anti-reflux security, (5) bubbler (containing the water), (6) Oil bath (maintained at temperature higher than that of the columns), (7) condenser, (8) Haake K thermostat ($\pm 0.1°C$), (9) gas-chromatograph (HP 5880) with dual thermal conductivity detector and integrator.

Instrumental device for dielectric measurements

Measurements of capacitance, C_d and C_0, and of the loss tangent, D_x, were carried out by means of a Low Frequency Impedance Analyser (HP 4192 A). The measuring cell consists of two concentric gold-plated brass cylinders (Fig. 4).

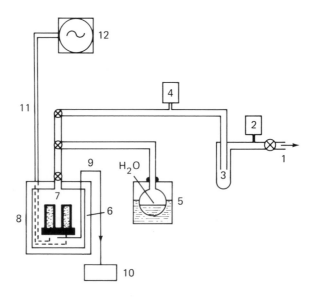

Fig. 4 — Block scheme of the dielectric measurement system. The different parts forming the measuring system are: (1) vacuum pumps, (2) Pirani gauge, (3) liquid nitrogen trap, (4) Penning gauge, (5) cold temperature source (thermostat) providing the desired relative humidity (its temperature varying from − 14°C to 67°C), (6) metal jar, (7) capacitance cell formed of coaxial cylinders, (8) oven, (9) Cu–Constantan thermocouple, (10) voltmeter (HP 3497A, for the data acquisition), (11) electric wires, (12) low frequency impedance analyser HP 4192A.

Materials and methods

Frontal chromatography

Column adsorbent: Fractosil® 5000 (E. Merck D-Darmstadt).

Column characteristics: length 36 cm
                        internal diameter 4.75 mm
                        external diameter 6.35 mm
                        amount of adsorbent about 4.69 g

Working temperatures: 40, 50, 60, 70°C (± 0.1°C)

Flow rate: 50 ml/min (± 1 ml/min)

Carrier gas: oxygen-free helium (purified through a molecular sieve: Katalysator R 3-11 (18820), Fluka, AG, CH-Buchs)

Packing was performed according to Tranchant's technique [11] and conditioned at 80°C for 48 hours under helium flow.

Dielectric measurements

All measurements were carried out on pure Fractosil® 5000 (E. Merck, Darmstadt, FRG) conditioned at relative humidities ranging from 3% to 90% and at 40, 50, 60 and 70°C.

Before the introduction of water vapour, the dielectric cell filled with Fractosil® 5000 (about 18.5 g) was outgassed at the isotherm temperature until a dynamic vacuum of 10^{-5} mmHg was recorded (at least 24 h). As for the water, it was outgassed separately by cooling it under vacuum (about 10^{-3} mmHg) with liquid nitrogen.

The desired relative humidities were obtained by regulating the temperature of the cold water source, which ranged from -14°C to 67°C (Fig. 4). Adsorption equilibrium was considered to have occurred once the capacitance C_d no longer changed with time. Preliminary runs showed that a minimum of a 12 h exposure of the sample to the cold water source was required to obtain reproducible capacitance readings. The surface coverage expressed in numbers of layers, θ, was deduced from the amount of adsorbed water and that of the monolayer determined by frontal gas-chromatography (eqn. (2)) and the BET model (eqn (5)).

RESULTS AND DISCUSSION

Water adsorption Isotherms on Fractosil® 5000
The water adsorption isotherms obtained by frontal GC and by elution GC are illustrated in Fig. 5. For low humidities, it is quite possible to establish

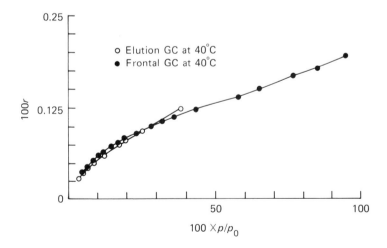

Fig. 5 — Water adsorption isotherm on Fractosil® 5000 at 40°C.

isotherms by elution chromatography. However, beyond approximately 40% relative humidity, the thermodynamic equilibrium becomes difficult to attain in elution GC and frontal GC appears to be a better method. The influence of the temperature on the quantity of adsorbed water is relatively small; the curves observed are affine and have the same type II shape according to the Brunauer–Deming–Deming–Teller classification [12] (Fig. 6). One of the problems is the differentiation of free- and of bound-water

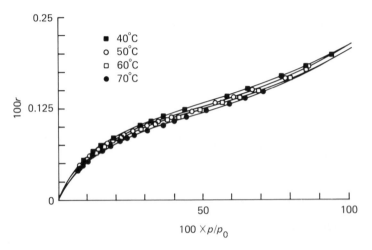

Fig. 6 — Water adsorption isotherms on Fractosil® 5000 at various temperatures.

and therefore the isotherms have been analysed according to the Hailwood–Horrobin model [5]. It appears that the quantity of bound-water remains constant beyond a monolayer (Fig. 7). Although the BET model is not quite appropriate (disregarding the adsorbate–adsorbate interactions beyond the monolayer) and that its corresponding treatment is questionable, it was nevertheless applied to calculate the amount of monolayer water and the specific surface areas of Fractosil® 5000, as a function of temperature using an average area of 10.6 Å^2 occupied by a water molecule. These specific surface areas correspond to the 3 m^2/g value obtained by nitrogen adsorption [13] and are almost independent of temperature (Table 1), at least in the 40–70°C range.

The isosteric enthalpy, ΔH_{iso} (Fig. 8), shows a minimum value (11.8 kcal/mol) at the monolayer, whereas the isosteric entropy, ΔS_{iso} (Fig. 9), shows a minimum value (-34 cal/mol K) beyond the monolayer at $\theta = 1.3$ for all isotherms in the 40–70°C range. As for the free energy, ΔG_{iso}, it decreases regularly with the surface coverage, θ (Fig. 10).

Dielectric isotherms of water vapour adsorbed on Fractosil® 5000

It is expected that the structural arrangement of the water is modified gradually with the growing thickness of the adsorbed layer. Therefore, at a fixed frequency, the dielectric constant ε' of the water/Fractosil® 5000

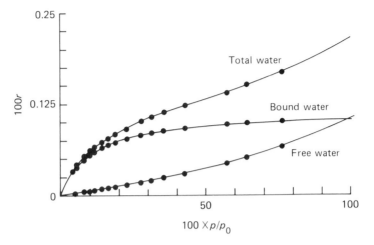

Fig. 7 — Adsorption isotherm of total-, bound- and free water on Fractosil® 5000 at
40°C.

Table 1 — Specific area, Σ_{H_2O}, relative quantity of water and net adsorption
heat, ΔH_{net} of the monolayer as a function of temperature

$T(°C)$	$\Sigma_{H_2O}(m^2/g)$	$10^4.r_m(g/g)$	$-\Delta H_{net}(kcal/mol)$
40	3.10 ± 0.03	8.7 ± 0.14	1.66 ± 0.02
50	2.98 ± 0.04	8.6 ± 0.11	1.66 ± 0.01
60	2.96 ± 0.04	8.4 ± 0.10	1.70 ± 0.02
70	2.86 ± 0.03	8.1 ± 0.09	1.76 ± 0.01

combined system increases with the coverage rate (Fig. 11). The changes in
dielectric constant, ε' (Fig. 11), reveal the existence of three apparently
different states of adsorbed water on Fractosil silica.

(a) The first layer of physically adsorbed water is immobile and presumably
doubly-hydrogen bonded to the underlying hydroxyl layer [16,17]. The
monolayer does not bring a significant change to the dielectric constant
ε', except for low frequencies for which a slight increase in ε' is recorded
(at $\theta \approx 0.6$). In fact the water molecules adsorbed in this layer are rigidly
held to the solid surface at fixed sites and they are therefore unable to
orient themselves in the alternating field, hence they cannot contribute
to the capacitance of the system.

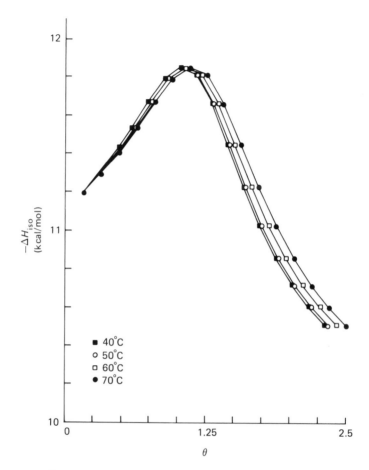

Fig. 8 — Variation of ΔH_{iso} as a function of θ for four temperatures.

(b) A second layer of water molecules, on the average singly hydrogen-bonded, is more mobile than the first layer. The dielectric constant ε' rises sharply and this increase is attributed to a higher ability of the adsorbed water molecules to respond to the alternative field current.

(c) Finally, after the second layer, the relative change in dielectric constant ε' seems to be constant. This attenuation in the growth of ε' indicates that the mobility of adsorbed water molecules has lessened.

The data for six different frequencies are illustrated in Fig. 11. For a given surface coverage, θ, the dielectric constant of the water/Fractosil® 5000 system decreases with an increase in the frequency.

From Table 2 or Fig. 12, it can be seen that the τ_0 value decreases when the amount of water adsorbed on Fractosil increases. At a $\theta < 0.6$ coverage, τ_0 is very large, this suggests that the adsorbed water is very tightly bound to the Fractosil surface. As more water molecules are absorbed, they become

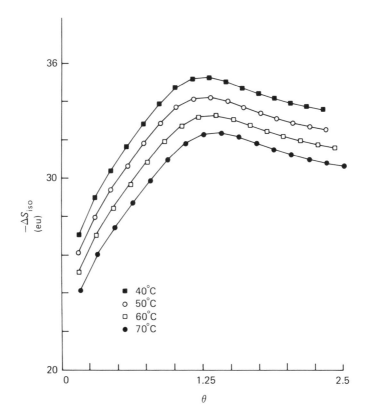

Fig. 9 — Variation of ΔS_{iso} as a function of θ for four temperatures.

mobile and tend to a structure having a relaxation time similar to that expected of ice (about 10^{-6} s at 298 K) at $\theta = 1.88$. The τ_{ice} value was calculated by Auty and Cole [18] by extrapolating the linear relationship between $\log \tau$ and $1/T$ (between 207.2 and 272.9 K), to 298 K. This value must be considered as the relaxation time which ice would have at 298 K, if ice could exist at that temperature.

At the monolayer, the relaxation time is inversely proportional to temperature (Table 3). It is therefore possible that τ_0 is an inverse function of both the surface coverage, θ, and the temperature T. The static dielectric constant, ε_s (Table 3), estimated from the Cole–Cole diagram, increases slightly with temperature.

The relaxation activation enthalpy, $\Delta H_{\varepsilon}^{\neq}$, is calculated from the temperature dependence of $\ln \nu_0$ according to equation (15). Like τ_0, $\Delta H_{\varepsilon}^{\neq}$ varies with the surface coverage, θ, and shows a maximum (7.3 kcal/mol) beyond the monolayer at $\theta = 1.3$ (Fig. 13); however, it does not vary significantly in the range of working temperatures.

As for the relaxation activation entropy, $\Delta S_{\varepsilon}^{\neq}$, it various with the surface

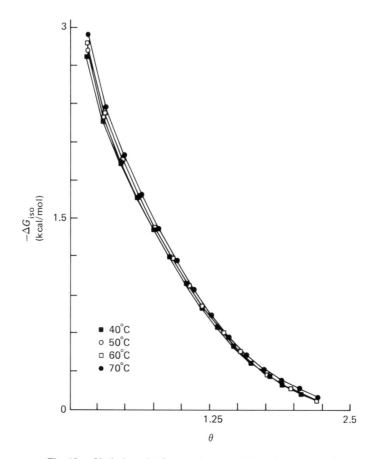

Fig. 10 — Variation of ΔG_{iso} as a function of θ for four temperatures.

coverage θ, and like $\Delta H_\varepsilon^{\neq}$, also has a maximum (-14 cal/mol K) beyond the monolayer at $\theta = 1.3$ (Fig. 14).

CONCLUSION

Although the general applicability for the determination of water adsorption isotherms on a large scale has still to be proven by other applications, the results obtained with Fractosil® 5000 show that frontal gas-chromatography could be an appropriate method for the fast determination of the amount of water adsorbed on a solid substance, and of the specific surface, Σ_{H_2O}, calculated according to BET.

The dielectric measurements appear to provide useful information related to the dynamic as well as to the molecular state of the water–excipient interface. The dielectric results obtained for Fractosil® 5000, such as the dielectric constant, the relaxation time, the relaxation activation

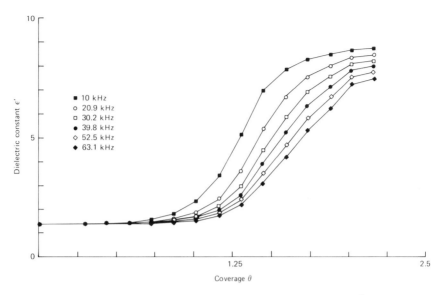

Fig. 11 — Dielectric constant, ε', of water vapour at 50°C on Fractosil® 5000 as a function of coverage at various frequencies.

Table 2 — Relaxation time, τ_0, static dielectric constant, ε_s, relaxation activation enthalpy, $\Delta H_\varepsilon^{\neq}$, and entropy, $\Delta S_\varepsilon^{\neq}$, as a function of the surface coverage, θ, at 50°C

θ	$\tau_0(s)$	ε_s	$\Delta H_\varepsilon^{\neq}$(kcal/mol)	$\Delta S_\varepsilon^{\neq}$(eu)
0.43	$6.5\ 10^{-3}$		1.3 ± 0.63	-44.6
0.58	$(2.6 \pm 0.13)\ 10^{-3}$	9.7 ± 0.30	2.6 ± 0.77	-38.9 ± 2.40
0.72	$(8.5 \pm 0.47)\ 10^{-4}$	9.9 ± 0.08	4.6 ± 0.83	-30.6 ± 2.58
0.87	$(3.0 \pm 0.03)\ 10^{-4}$	9.9 ± 0.04	6.0 ± 0.93	-24.0 ± 2.88
1.01	$(1.1 \pm 0.02)\ 10^{-4}$	9.7 ± 0.01	6.4 ± 1.07	-20.8 ± 3.32
1.16	$(4.4 \pm 0.14)\ 10^{-5}$	9.7 ± 0.01	7.3 ± 1.17	-16.3 ± 3.63
1.30	$(1.8 \pm 0.06)\ 10^{-5}$	9.7 ± 0.01	7.3 ± 1.37	-14.3 ± 4.26
1.44	$(7.9 \pm 0.31)\ 10^{-6}$	9.6 ± 0.01	5.8 ± 1.11	-17.3 ± 3.45
1.59	$(4.3 \pm 0.16)\ 10^{-6}$	9.6 ± 0.01	4.6 ± 1.02	-20.1 ± 3.17
1.73	$(2.7 \pm 0.12)\ 10^{-6}$	9.6 ± 0.01	3.9 ± 1.40	-21.3 ± 4.34
1.88	$(1.8 \pm 0.07)\ 10^{-6}$	9.6 ± 0.01	1.7 ± 0.96	-27.3 ± 2.98

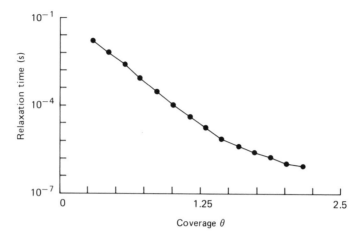

Fig. 12 — Relaxation time of adsorbed water vapour on Fractosil® 5000 at 50°C as a function of the surface coverage.

Table 3 — Monolayer relaxation time, τ_0, static dielectric constant, ε_s, relaxation activation enthalpy, $\Delta H_\varepsilon^{\neq}$, and entropy, $\Delta S_\varepsilon^{\neq}$, as a function of temperature

$T(°C)$	$10^5 \cdot \tau_0$ (s)	ε_s	$\Delta H_\varepsilon^{\neq}$(kcal/mol)	$\Delta S_\varepsilon^{\neq}$(eu)
40	12.8 ± 0.03	9.7 ± 0.01	6.4 ± 1.07	− 20.3 ± 3.42
50	11.1 ± 0.02	9.7 ± 0.01	6.4 ± 1.07	− 20.8 ± 3.32
60	6.8 ± 0.27	9.9 ± 0.02	6.4 ± 1.07	− 20.5 ± 3.22
70	5.0 ± 0.31	10.0 ± 0.03	6.4 ± 1.07	− 20.8 ± 3.13

enthalpy and entropy suggest that three distinct adsorption states exist for water adsorbed on Fractosil® 5000: an immobile first layer, a second layer more mobile than the first and finally ordered layers. Although more work is needed to draw valuable conclusions, it seems that the best qualitative description of the water–excipient system is given by the water relaxation time in conjunction with the amount of adsorbed water. The latter is more sensitive than any other related dielectric or thermodynamic parameter drawn from the same experimental results.

ACKNOWLEDGEMENTS

The authors gratefully acknowledge the partial support of the Swiss National Foundation.

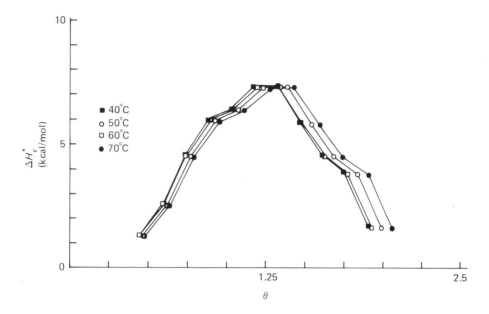

Fig. 13 — Relaxation activation enthalpy as a function of coverage.

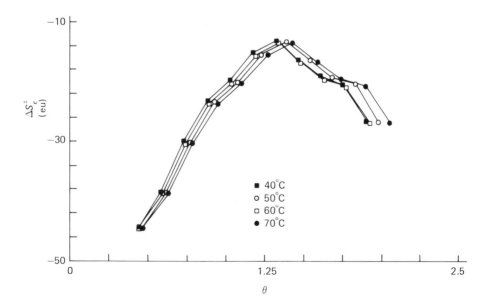

Fig. 14 — Relaxation activation entropy as a function of coverage.

REFERENCES

[1] J. T. Carstensen, in *Pharmaceutics of Solids and Solid Dosage Form,* John Wiley & Sons, New York, pp 194–202 (1977).

[2] J. B. Mielck and H. Rabach, *Acta Pharm. Technol.,* **30**, 33 (1984).

[3] J. Chauchard, B. Chabert, H. Etienne and J. P. Soulier, *Ann. Chim.,* **7**, 103–112 (1972).

[4] S. Brunauer, P. H. Emmett and E. Teller, *J. Am. Chem. Soc.,* **60**, 309, (1938).

[5] A. J. Hailwood and S. Horrobin, *Trans. Faraday Soc.,* **42-B**, 84 (1946).

[6] D. A. King and C. A. Woodruff, in *The Chemical Physics of Solid Surfaces and Heterogeneous Catalysis,* vol. 2, Elsevier, Amsterdam, Oxford, New York, pp. 14–16 (1983).

[7] P. Debye, in *Polar Molecules,* Dover Publications, New York, p. 89 (1929).

[8] K. S. Cole and R. H. Cole, *J. Chem. Phys.,* **9**, 341–351 (1941).

[9] S. Glasstone, K. J. Laidler and H. Eyring, in *Theory of Rate Processes,* McGraw-Hill Book Company, New York, p. 548 (1941).

[10] Saint-Yrieix Alain, *Bull. Soc. Chim. de France,* **10**, 3433 (1971).

[11] J. Tranchant, in *Manual Pratique de Chromatographie en Phase Gazeuse,* 3ème edn, Masson, Paris, pp. 152–182 (1982).

[12] S. Brunauer, L. S. Deming, W. S. Deming and E. Teller, *J. Am. Chem. Soc.,* **62**, 1723 (1940).

[13] Reagenzien Merck, 1980, p. 19, E. Merck Postfach 4119, D-6100 Darmstadt.

[14] *Handbook of Chemistry and Physics,* Ed. The Chemical Rubber Co., Cleveland, Ohio, p. D109 (1968).

[15] D. W. Marquardt, *J. Soc. Indust. and Appl. Math.,* **2**, pp. 431–441 (1963).

[16] A. V. Kiselev in *Structure and Properties of Porous Materials,* D. H. Everett and F. S. Stone (eds), Academic Press, New York, p. 195 (1958).

[17] A. C. Zettlemoyer, R. D. Iyengar and P. Scheidt, *J. Colloid Interface Sci.,* **22**, 172 (1966).

[18] R. P. Auty and R. H. Cole, *J. Chem. Phys.,* **20**, 1309 (1952).

Index